The Science Behind Nutrition

The Definitive Guide to Debunking Diet Myths and Practicing Responsible Eating for Optimal Health and Happiness

BY
ADEEL ANJUM

CONTENTS

INTRODUCTION

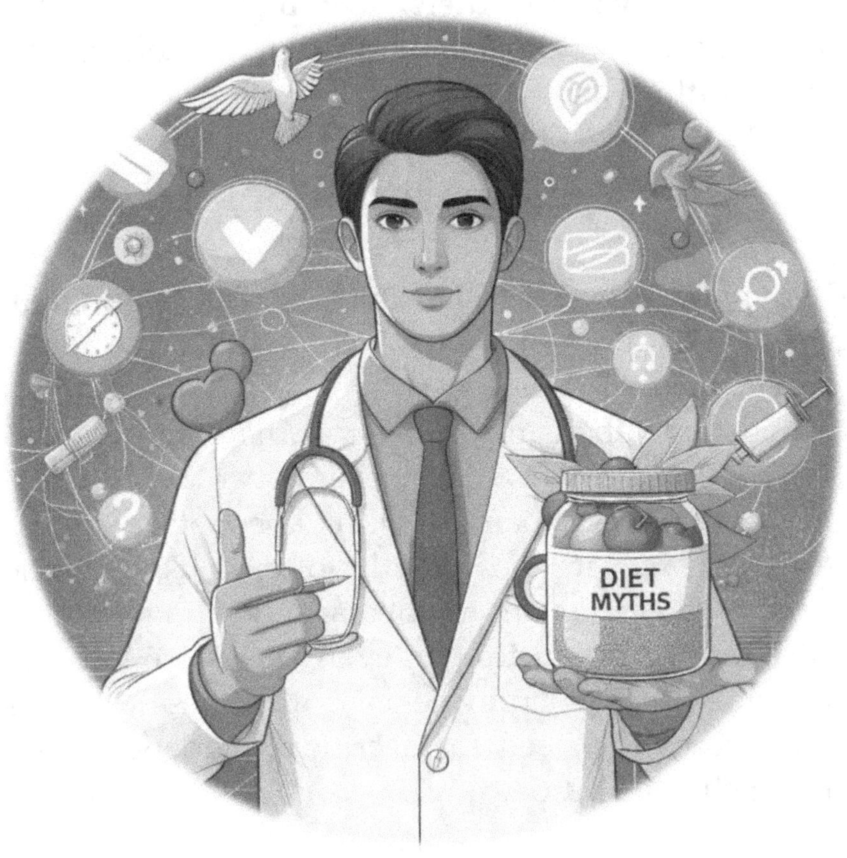

In today's world, the topic of nutrition is saturated with a vast array of conflicting information and numerous diet myths. From celebrity-endorsed weight loss plans to fad diets that promise miraculous results, it can be incredibly challenging to distinguish fact from fiction. This confusion is compounded by the rapid dissemination of information via social media, where influencers and self-proclaimed experts often present their opinions as established truths. Consequently, many people find themselves caught in a cycle of trying and abandoning various diets, leading to frustration, misinformation, and often detrimental effects on their health.

The Problem with Diet Myths

Diet myths are pervasive and can be remarkably persuasive. Common myths include ideas like "carbs are the enemy," "you must eat small, frequent meals to boost metabolism," or "detox diets can cleanse your body of toxins." Such claims can be enticing, especially when paired with anecdotal success stories. However, these myths often lack scientific backing and can result in unbalanced eating patterns, nutritional deficiencies, or even disordered eating behaviors. The prevalence of these myths underscores the need for a critical, evidence-based approach to nutrition.

The Importance of Evidence-Based, Personalized Eating

Optimal health and well-being are best achieved through evidence-based, personalized eating practices. Unlike one-size-fits-all diets, which often fail to address individual needs and preferences, a personalized approach considers unique factors such as genetics, lifestyle, health conditions, and personal goals. Scientific research supports the notion that no single diet is universally effective; rather, the best dietary practices are those tailored to fit the specific needs of each person. This approach not only enhances physical health but also promotes a positive relationship with food, reducing the stress and guilt often associated with eating.

Roadmap and Key Takeaways

This book, "The Science Behind Nutrition: The Definitive Guide to Debunking Diet Myths and Practicing Responsible Eating for Optimal Health and Happiness," aims to provide readers with a comprehensive understanding of nutrition based on the latest scientific evidence. Each chapter will delve into specific aspects of diet and nutrition, debunking common myths and offering practical, actionable advice for adopting healthier eating habits.

Key Takeaways:

- Understanding Nutrition Fundamentals: Gain a solid foundation in nutritional science, including macronutrients, micronutrients, and the role of various food groups.
- Debunking Common Diet Myths: Identify and critically analyze popular diet myths, understanding the science (or lack thereof) behind them.

- Personalized Nutrition: Learn how to tailor dietary choices to individual needs, considering factors such as age, gender, activity level, and health conditions.
- Practical Eating Strategies: Discover practical tips and strategies for making healthier food choices, meal planning, and maintaining a balanced diet.
- Promoting a Positive Relationship with Food: Foster a healthier, more mindful approach to eating that emphasizes enjoyment and well-being over restriction and guilt.

Throughout the book, we will emphasize the importance of informed decision-making and provide tools to help readers navigate the complex landscape of nutrition. By the end of this guide, you will be equipped with the knowledge and confidence to make dietary choices that enhance your health and happiness.

Let's embark on this journey to demystify nutrition and empower ourselves with the truth about what we eat. The path to optimal health and happiness starts with understanding the science behind nutrition and making informed, responsible eating choices.

Part 1: Understanding the Fundamentals of Nutrition

Chapter 01

Macronutrients: The Building Blocks of Your Diet

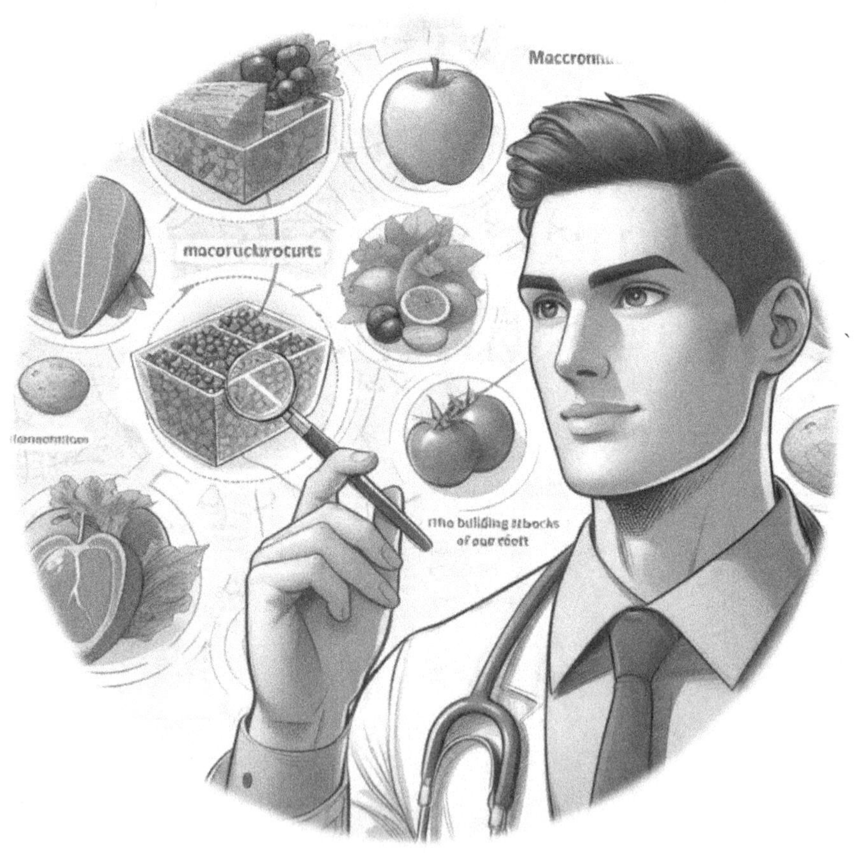

Understanding the fundamentals of nutrition begins with grasping the essential components that constitute our diet: macronutrients. These vital nutrients—carbohydrates, proteins, and fats—are required in relatively large amounts and play critical roles in maintaining our overall health. Each macronutrient has unique functions and contributions to the body's energy supply, growth, and repair processes. In this chapter, we will explore these building blocks in detail, debunk common myths, and provide actionable steps to determine your individual macronutrient needs.

What are Macronutrients?

Macronutrients are the nutrients our bodies need in large quantities to function optimally. Unlike micronutrients, which are needed in smaller amounts (such as vitamins and minerals), macronutrients provide the energy necessary for daily activities and bodily functions. There are three primary types of macronutrients:

- Carbohydrates
- Proteins
- Fats

Each macronutrient serves specific roles and is vital for maintaining health and supporting bodily functions.

Carbohydrates: The Body's Primary Energy Source

Carbohydrates are often misunderstood and misrepresented in the realm of diet myths. They are the body's main source of energy, particularly for the brain and muscles during exercise.

Types of Carbohydrates:

1. Simple Carbohydrates: These are quickly digested and provide rapid energy. They include sugars found in fruits (fructose), dairy (lactose), and table sugar (sucrose). While naturally occurring sugars in whole foods are beneficial, added sugars in processed foods can lead to blood sugar spikes and crashes.

2. Complex Carbohydrates: These consist of long chains of sugar molecules and are found in foods such as whole grains, legumes, and vegetables. They are digested more slowly, providing a steady release of energy and maintaining stable blood sugar levels.

Impact on Blood Sugar:

Carbohydrates affect blood sugar levels differently depending on their type and the presence of fiber. Simple carbohydrates can cause quick spikes in blood sugar, leading to a rapid release of insulin. In contrast, complex carbohydrates, especially those high in fiber, result in a slower, more gradual increase in blood sugar, promoting sustained energy levels and better satiety.

Protein: Building and Repairing Tissues

Protein is crucial for the growth, repair, and maintenance of tissues in the body. It is composed of amino acids, some of which are essential, meaning they must be obtained through the diet as the body cannot produce them.

Roles of Protein:

- Muscle Repair and Growth: Protein is vital for repairing and building muscles, especially after exercise.
- Enzyme and Hormone Production: Proteins are necessary for creating enzymes and hormones that regulate bodily functions.
- Immune Function: Proteins play a key role in producing antibodies and supporting the immune system.

Sources of Protein:

Proteins can be obtained from both animal and plant sources. Animal proteins, such as meat, poultry, fish, eggs, and dairy, are complete proteins, meaning they contain all essential amino acids. Plant-based proteins, such as beans, lentils, nuts, seeds, and soy products, can also provide adequate protein but may need to be combined to ensure all essential amino acids are consumed.

Fats: Essential for Hormone Production and Satiety

Fats often get a bad reputation, but they are essential for numerous bodily functions. They provide a concentrated source of energy, support cell growth, protect organs, and help with nutrient absorption.

Types of Fats:

1. Saturated Fats: Typically found in animal products and some tropical oils, these fats have been historically linked to heart disease. However, recent research suggests that the relationship is more complex, and moderate consumption of saturated fats may not be as harmful as once thought.

2. Unsaturated Fats: These are further divided into:

   - Monounsaturated Fats: Found in olive oil, avocados, and nuts, they are known for their heart health benefits.
   - Polyunsaturated Fats: These include omega-3 and omega-6 fatty acids, found in fatty fish, flaxseeds, and walnuts. Omega-3s, in

particular, are anti-inflammatory and support brain health.

3. Trans Fats: Artificial trans fats, found in some processed foods, are harmful and have been linked to increased heart disease risk. It's best to avoid these entirely.

Role in Hormone Production and Satiety:

Healthy fats are critical for hormone production, including sex hormones like estrogen and testosterone. They also help regulate satiety by slowing the digestion process, making you feel fuller for longer and preventing overeating.

Debunking Myths Surrounding "Good" and "Bad" Fats

One of the most persistent diet myths is the notion of "good" and "bad" fats. While it is true that some fats are healthier than others, the key is understanding their roles and incorporating them appropriately into your diet.

Myth: "All fats are bad and should be avoided."
Fact: Healthy fats are essential for bodily functions and should be included in a balanced diet. Avoiding fats entirely can lead to nutrient deficiencies and hormonal imbalances.

Myth: "Saturated fats are the primary cause of heart disease."
Fact: Recent studies indicate that the link between saturated fats and heart disease is not as clear-cut. Moderation is key, and the overall quality of the diet matters more.

Myth: "Low-fat diets are the best for weight loss."
Fact: Low-fat diets can be counterproductive as they often replace fats with refined carbohydrates, leading to blood sugar spikes and increased hunger. Balanced diets with healthy fats can be more effective for weight management.

Action Steps: Identifying Your Individual Macronutrient Needs

To determine your individual macronutrient needs, consider factors such as age, gender, activity level, and specific health goals. Here are some actionable steps to help you personalize your macronutrient intake:

1. **Calculate Your Basal Metabolic Rate (BMR):** This is the number of calories your body needs at rest. Online calculators can help you estimate this based on your age, weight, height, and gender.

2. **Determine Your Total Daily Energy Expenditure (TDEE):** Multiply your BMR by an

activity factor that reflects your lifestyle (sedentary, lightly active, moderately active, very active).

3. **Set Your Macronutrient Ratios:** Based on your TDEE and health goals, allocate a percentage of your calories to each macronutrient:

    - Carbohydrates: Typically 45-65% of total calories.
    - Proteins: Typically 10-35% of total calories.
    - Fats: Typically 20-35% of total calories.

4. **Adjust Based on Goals:**

    - Weight Loss: Focus on a slight caloric deficit while ensuring adequate protein to preserve muscle mass.
    - Muscle Gain: Aim for a caloric surplus with increased protein intake to support muscle repair and growth.
    - Maintenance: Balance your intake to maintain current weight and support overall health.

5. **Monitor and Adjust:** Regularly assess your energy levels, performance, and overall well-being. Adjust your macronutrient intake as needed to meet your changing goals and needs.

Conclusion

Understanding macronutrients and their roles in the body is fundamental to making informed dietary choices. Carbohydrates, proteins, and fats each contribute uniquely to our health and well-being. By debunking myths and focusing on personalized nutrition, you can develop a balanced diet that supports your individual needs and promotes optimal health. Remember, the goal is not to follow a rigid set of rules but to make informed, flexible choices that fit your lifestyle and goals.

Chapter 02

Micronutrients: The Powerhouse Players

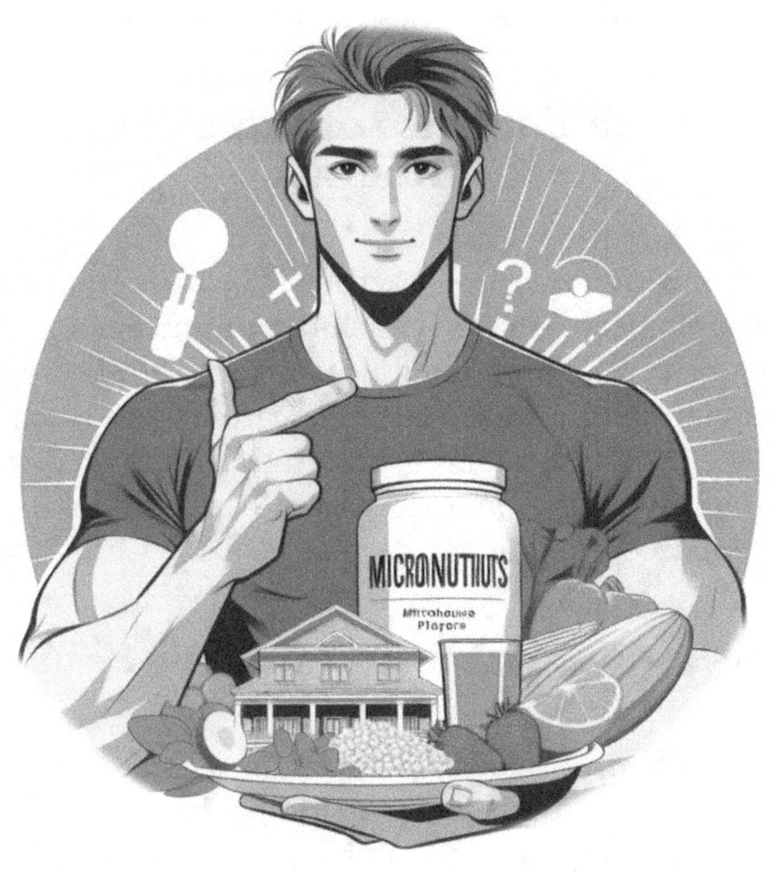

While macronutrients provide the bulk of our dietary needs and energy, micronutrients—vitamins and minerals—are the unsung heroes that ensure our bodies function smoothly. Even though they are required in smaller quantities, their impact on health is profound. This chapter delves into the vital roles that vitamins and minerals play, debunks common myths, and offers actionable steps to ensure you get an adequate intake of these essential nutrients.

The Importance of Vitamins and Minerals

Micronutrients are crucial for numerous physiological processes, including immune function, energy production, bone health, and cellular repair. Deficiencies in these nutrients can lead to a variety of health issues, ranging from fatigue and weakened immunity to more severe conditions like osteoporosis and anemia.

Essential Vitamins and Their Sources

Vitamins are organic compounds that are essential for normal growth and nutrition. They are divided into two categories: fat-soluble and water-soluble.

Fat-Soluble Vitamins

1. Vitamin A: Important for vision, immune function, and skin health.

- Sources: Carrots, sweet potatoes, spinach, and liver.

2. Vitamin D: Essential for bone health as it helps in calcium absorption. Also supports immune function.

- Sources: Sunlight exposure, fortified dairy products, fatty fish, and egg yolks.

3. Vitamin E: Acts as an antioxidant, protecting cells from damage. It also supports immune function.

- Sources: Nuts, seeds, spinach, and broccoli.

4. Vitamin K: Necessary for blood clotting and bone health.

- Sources: Leafy greens like kale and spinach, broccoli, and Brussels sprouts.

Water-Soluble Vitamins

1. Vitamin C: Vital for the growth and repair of tissues, it also acts as an antioxidant.

- Sources: Citrus fruits, strawberries, bell peppers, and broccoli.

2. B Vitamins: This group of vitamins (including B1,

B2, B3, B6, B12, folate, and biotin) is crucial for energy production, brain function, and cell metabolism.

- Sources: Whole grains, meat, eggs, dairy products, legumes, seeds, and leafy greens.

Essential Minerals and Their Roles

Minerals are inorganic elements that play various roles in maintaining health. Here are some key minerals and their functions:

1. Calcium: Essential for strong bones and teeth, muscle function, and nerve signaling.
- Sources: Dairy products, leafy greens, tofu, and fortified plant milks.

2. Magnesium: Involved in over 300 biochemical reactions, including energy production, muscle function, and nerve function.
- Sources: Nuts, seeds, whole grains, and green leafy vegetables.

3. Iron: Critical for the production of hemoglobin, which carries oxygen in the blood.
- Sources: Red meat, poultry, beans, lentils, fortified cereals, and spinach.

4. Potassium: Helps regulate fluid balance, muscle

contractions, and nerve signals.

- Sources: Bananas, oranges, potatoes, and spinach.

5. Zinc: Supports immune function, wound healing, and DNA synthesis.

- Sources: Meat, shellfish, dairy, nuts, and legumes.

Debunking Myths Surrounding Megadosing Vitamins and Supplements

A common misconception is that if some vitamins are good, more must be better. This has led to the popularity of megadosing—taking vitamins in quantities significantly higher than the recommended daily allowance (RDA). However, this practice can be harmful rather than beneficial.

Myth: "Megadosing vitamins can prevent illness and boost health."

Fact: While certain vitamins in large doses might have therapeutic uses (e.g., vitamin C for colds), routinely taking high doses can cause toxicity and adverse effects. For example, excessive vitamin A can lead to liver damage, and too much vitamin D can result in hypercalcemia, which affects the heart and kidneys.

Myth: "Supplements can replace a balanced diet."
Fact: Supplements should not replace whole foods. Whole foods contain a complex matrix of nutrients and phytochemicals that work synergistically. Isolated nutrients in supplements do not provide the same benefits and can sometimes lead to imbalances or nutrient competition in the body.

The Importance of a Balanced Diet for Micronutrient Sufficiency

A balanced diet rich in a variety of foods is the best way to ensure adequate micronutrient intake. This approach helps prevent deficiencies and promotes overall health. Foods in their natural state provide a range of nutrients that supplements cannot fully replicate.

Action Steps: Exploring Colorful Fruits and Vegetables to Increase Micronutrient Intake

To boost your intake of vitamins and minerals, focus on incorporating a wide variety of colorful fruits and vegetables into your diet. Here are some practical tips:

1. Eat the Rainbow: Include fruits and vegetables of different colors in your meals. Each color often

represents different types of nutrients. For example:

- Red: Tomatoes, strawberries, and red peppers (rich in antioxidants like lycopene and vitamin C).
- Orange/Yellow: Carrots, sweet potatoes, and oranges (high in beta-carotene and vitamin C).
- Green: Spinach, kale, and broccoli (packed with vitamins K, C, and folate).
- Blue/Purple: Blueberries, eggplants, and purple cabbage (contain anthocyanins and vitamin C).

2. Smoothies and Salads: Blend fruits and vegetables into smoothies for a nutrient-dense breakfast or snack. Create vibrant salads with a variety of ingredients to ensure a broad spectrum of vitamins and minerals.

3. Seasonal Eating: Opt for seasonal produce, which is often fresher and more nutrient-dense. Visit local farmers' markets to explore new fruits and vegetables.

4. Cooking Methods: Use cooking methods that preserve nutrients, such as steaming, roasting, or lightly sautéing. Avoid overcooking vegetables, which can deplete their vitamin content.

5. Snacking Smart: Keep a supply of fruits, vegetable sticks, and nuts for convenient, healthy snacks. This can help you avoid processed foods that are often low in essential nutrients.

Conclusion

Micronutrients, though needed in smaller amounts, are indispensable to our health. Vitamins and minerals support a wide range of bodily functions, and a deficiency in any of them can lead to significant health problems. By understanding the importance of these nutrients, debunking myths about supplementation, and focusing on a balanced diet rich in colorful fruits and vegetables, you can ensure you meet your daily micronutrient needs. Embracing these practices will pave the way for improved health and vitality, helping you feel your best every day.

Chapter 03

Digestion and Gut Health: The Key to Overall Wellbeing

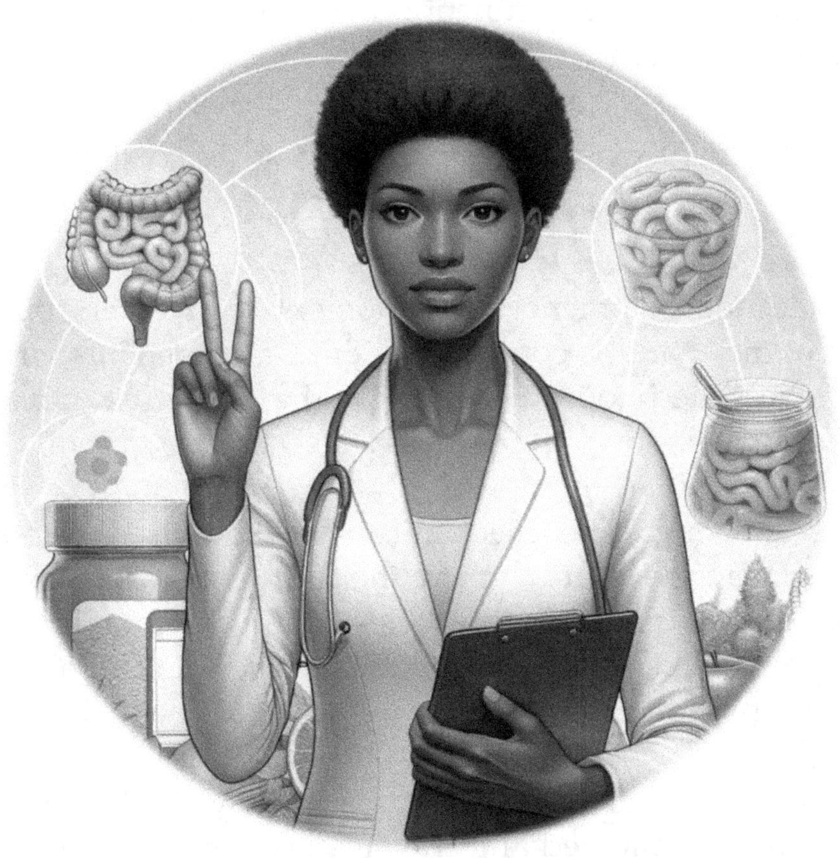

Digestion is a remarkably intricate process, serving as the gateway through which the food we eat is broken down, absorbed, and utilized by our bodies. Beyond its fundamental role in nutrient extraction, digestion is intricately connected to various aspects of health, particularly through its relationship with the gut microbiome. In this comprehensive exploration, we will delve into the complexities of digestion, the profound influence of gut health on overall wellbeing, and actionable strategies to optimize digestive function and nurture a thriving gut microbiome.

The Digestive Process: A Journey Through the Gut

Digestion commences the moment food enters our mouths and continues on a meticulously orchestrated journey through the digestive tract. Let's break down the process step by step:

1. Chewing: The mechanical breakdown of food begins in the mouth, where the teeth grind and mash food into smaller particles. Saliva, containing enzymes like amylase, initiates the digestion of carbohydrates.

2. Swallowing: Once adequately chewed, the food bolus is swallowed and travels down the esophagus to the stomach through peristaltic contractions.

3. Stomach: In the stomach, gastric juices containing hydrochloric acid and pepsin further break down food into a semi-liquid substance called chyme. Proteins are primarily digested here.

4. Small Intestine: The majority of nutrient absorption occurs in the small intestine, where enzymes from the pancreas and bile from the liver aid in the digestion of carbohydrates, fats, and proteins. Nutrients are absorbed through the intestinal wall into the bloodstream.

5. Large Intestine: Any remaining indigestible material passes into the large intestine, where water and electrolytes are reabsorbed, and beneficial bacteria in the gut microbiome ferment fiber and produce short-chain fatty acids.

6. Elimination: Finally, waste material is formed into stool and expelled from the body through the rectum and anus.

The Gut Microbiome: Your Body's Ecosystem

The gut microbiome is a bustling community of trillions of microorganisms residing in the gastrointestinal tract, collectively weighing around 2 kilograms. This diverse ecosystem comprises bacteria, fungi, viruses, and other microbes, each playing a unique role in gut health and overall wellbeing.

Impact on Digestion: Certain bacteria in the gut produce enzymes that aid in the breakdown of complex carbohydrates and fibers, facilitating their digestion and absorption. Additionally, short-chain fatty acids produced by gut bacteria serve as an energy source for colon cells and play a role in reducing inflammation.

Immunity: The gut microbiome interacts closely with the immune system, influencing the development and function of immune cells and helping to distinguish between harmful pathogens and beneficial bacteria. A balanced microbiome is essential for maintaining immune homeostasis and protecting against infections.

Mood Regulation: The gut-brain axis facilitates bidirectional communication between the gut and the brain, allowing for the exchange of signals that influence mood, behavior, and cognitive function. Emerging research suggests that alterations in the gut microbiome may be linked to mood disorders such as depression and anxiety.

Prebiotics and Probiotics: Nurturing Your Gut Garden

Maintaining a healthy gut microbiome is key to supporting optimal digestion and overall health.

Prebiotics and probiotics are two essential components of gut health management:

Prebiotics: These indigestible fibers serve as food for beneficial bacteria in the gut, promoting their growth and activity. Examples of prebiotic-rich foods include garlic, onions, leeks, asparagus, bananas, oats, and Jerusalem artichokes.

Probiotics: Live microorganisms that confer health benefits when consumed in adequate amounts. Probiotic-rich foods include yogurt, kefir, sauerkraut, kimchi, miso, tempeh, and kombucha. These foods introduce beneficial bacteria into the gut, helping to maintain microbial balance and support digestive health.

Debunking Myths Surrounding Cleanses and Detox Diets

Cleanses and detox diets have gained popularity in recent years, often touted as a means to cleanse the body of toxins, promote weight loss, and enhance overall health. However, many of these claims lack scientific evidence and may even pose risks to health:

Myth: "Detox diets cleanse the body of toxins."
Fact: The body possesses its own highly efficient detoxification mechanisms, primarily the liver and kidneys, which filter and eliminate toxins from the body. Extreme detox diets or cleanses may disrupt

normal bodily functions and lead to nutrient deficiencies.

Myth: "Cleanses promote weight loss."
Fact: While some cleanses may result in temporary weight loss due to water weight and calorie restriction, this weight loss is not sustainable in the long term. Cleanses that severely restrict calories can slow metabolism and lead to muscle loss, undermining overall health.

Mindful Eating and Stress Management for Digestive Harmony

In addition to dietary interventions, mindful eating practices and stress management techniques can profoundly impact digestive health:

Mindful Eating: Slowing down and savoring each bite, paying attention to hunger and fullness cues, and minimizing distractions during meals can promote better digestion and nutrient absorption. Chewing food thoroughly and allowing time for proper digestion reduces the likelihood of digestive discomfort such as bloating and indigestion.

Stress Management: Chronic stress can impair digestion by triggering the release of stress hormones like cortisol, which can disrupt normal digestive processes and exacerbate symptoms of conditions like irritable bowel syndrome (IBS). Stress management techniques such as meditation, deep breathing exercises, yoga, and regular physical activity can help reduce stress levels and promote digestive harmony.

Action Steps: Nourishing Your Gut for Optimal Health

To cultivate a thriving gut microbiome and support optimal digestion, consider incorporating the following action steps into your daily routine:

1. Embrace Fermented Foods: Introduce probiotic-rich foods like yogurt, kefir, kimchi, sauerkraut, miso, tempeh, and kombucha into your diet regularly to promote microbial diversity and gut health.

2. Prioritize Prebiotics: Consume a variety of prebiotic-rich foods such as garlic, onions, leeks, asparagus, bananas, oats, and Jerusalem artichokes to nourish beneficial bacteria in the gut and enhance their activity.

3. Foster Fiber Intake: Increase your consumption of fiber-rich foods such as fruits, vegetables, legumes, whole grains, nuts, and seeds to support regular bowel movements, promote satiety, and provide fuel for gut bacteria.

4. Practice Mindful Eating: Create a peaceful eating

environment free from distractions, chew food thoroughly, and listen to your body's hunger and fullness cues to optimize digestion and nutrient absorption.

5. Manage Stress: Incorporate stress-reduction techniques such as meditation, deep breathing exercises, yoga, regular physical activity, and spending time in nature to minimize the impact of stress on digestive health.

Conclusion: Nurturing Your Gut, Nourishing Your Health

In conclusion, digestion and gut health are foundational pillars of overall wellbeing, influencing everything from nutrient absorption to immune function and mood regulation. By understanding the intricacies of the digestive process, nurturing a diverse and balanced gut microbiome, and adopting mindful eating practices and stress management techniques, you can optimize digestive function and support vibrant health from within. Incorporating probiotic-rich fermented foods, prebiotic-rich plant foods, and fiber into your diet can provide essential nutrients and promote the growth of beneficial gut bacteria. By prioritizing gut health, you can enhance your overall vitality and wellbeing, allowing you to thrive and flourish in every aspect of life.

Chapter 04

Fueling Your Body for Energy and Performance

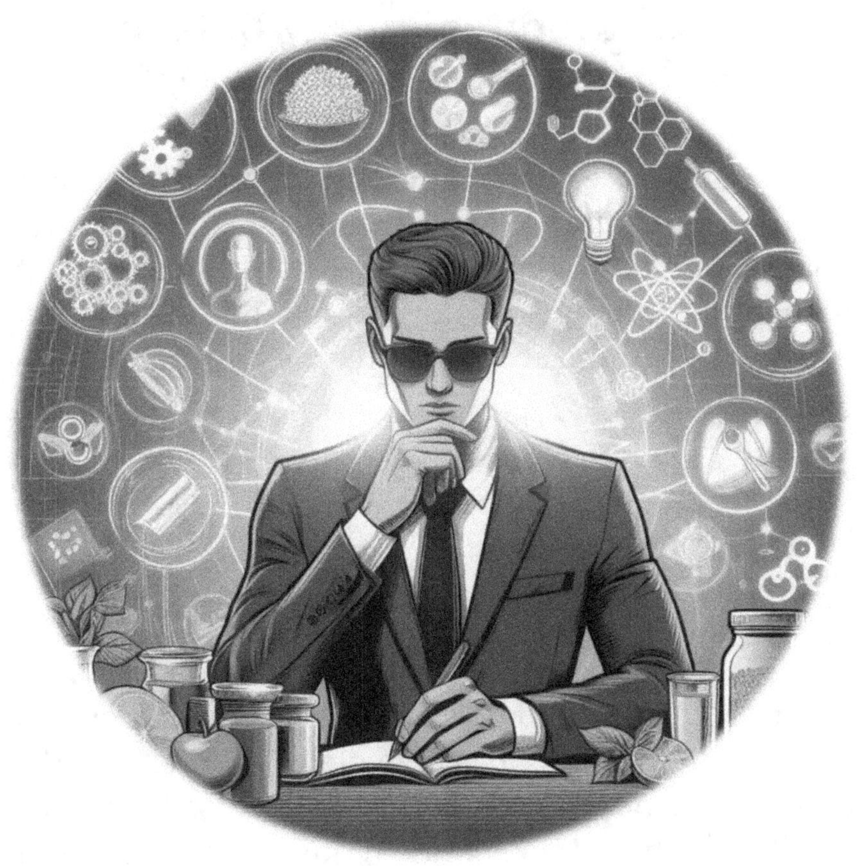

Optimizing nutrition is crucial for fueling your body, enhancing performance, and supporting overall vitality. In this chapter, we will delve into the principles of energy balance, the significance of macronutrient ratios, pre and post-workout nutrition strategies, debunking myths surrounding fad diets, emphasizing hydration, and providing actionable steps to ensure you're adequately fueling your body for energy and peak performance.

Understanding Energy Balance: Calories In vs. Calories Out

Energy balance is the foundation of weight management and overall health. It refers to the relationship between the calories consumed through food and beverages (calories in) and the calories expended through metabolism and physical activity (calories out).

Calories In: The energy derived from the foods and beverages you consume provides the fuel necessary for bodily functions, physical activity, and metabolism.

Calories Out: This encompasses the energy expended through basal metabolic rate (BMR), physical activity, and the thermic effect of food (TEF), which is the energy required for digestion, absorption, and metabolism of nutrients.

Maintaining a balance between calories consumed and calories expended is essential for weight maintenance, weight loss, or weight gain, depending on individual goals and needs.

Importance of Macronutrient Ratios for Different Activity Levels

The composition of your diet, particularly the ratio of macronutrients—carbohydrates, proteins, and fats—plays a pivotal role in supporting different activity levels and performance goals.

Carbohydrates: As the body's primary source of energy, carbohydrates are crucial for fueling high-intensity exercise and replenishing glycogen stores. Athletes and individuals engaged in intense physical activity may benefit from higher carbohydrate intake to sustain performance and prevent fatigue.

Proteins: Protein is essential for muscle repair, growth, and recovery, particularly for individuals engaging in resistance training or endurance exercise. Adequate protein intake supports muscle maintenance and repair, aiding in recovery and adaptation to exercise.

Fats: While often overlooked in sports nutrition, fats play a vital role in providing sustained energy, supporting hormone production, and aiding in the absorption of fat-soluble vitamins. Including healthy fats in your diet can enhance satiety and provide a source of long-lasting energy for endurance activities.

Pre-Workout and Post-Workout Nutrition for Optimal Performance

Pre-Workout Nutrition: Fueling your body adequately before exercise can enhance performance and optimize energy levels. Aim to consume a balanced meal or snack containing carbohydrates, protein, and a small amount of fat 1-2 hours before exercise to provide sustained energy and support muscle function.

Post-Workout Nutrition: Following exercise, prioritize replenishing glycogen stores, repairing muscle tissue, and promoting recovery by consuming a combination of carbohydrates and protein within 30-60 minutes post-workout. This helps facilitate muscle glycogen resynthesis, reduces muscle breakdown, and promotes muscle repair and growth.

Debunking Myths Surrounding Fad Diets and Extreme Calorie Restriction

In the pursuit of optimal performance and physique, many individuals are drawn to fad diets and extreme calorie restriction. However, these approaches often yield temporary results and can have detrimental effects on health and performance.

Myth: "Extreme calorie restriction leads to rapid weight loss and improved performance."
Fact: Severe calorie restriction can lead to nutrient deficiencies, muscle loss, decreased energy levels, and impaired performance. Sustainable weight loss and performance improvements are best achieved through gradual, balanced approaches that prioritize adequate nutrition and fueling for activity.

Myth: "Fad diets offer a quick fix for achieving optimal performance."
Fact: Fad diets typically involve restrictive eating patterns that are unsustainable in the long term and may lack essential nutrients needed for optimal performance and overall health. Instead of focusing on short-term fixes, prioritize balanced, nutrient-dense meals that support your energy needs and performance goals.

Importance of Hydration for Energy Levels and Overall Health

Hydration is often overlooked but is essential for maintaining optimal energy levels, supporting physiological functions, and sustaining performance, particularly during exercise.

Fluid Balance: Water plays a critical role in

regulating body temperature, transporting nutrients, and removing waste products from the body. Even mild dehydration can impair physical and cognitive performance, leading to fatigue, reduced endurance, and impaired concentration.

Electrolyte Balance: During prolonged or intense exercise, electrolytes such as sodium, potassium, and magnesium are lost through sweat and must be replenished to maintain proper hydration and electrolyte balance. Consuming electrolyte-rich fluids or sports drinks can help replace lost fluids and electrolytes during exercise.

Action Steps: Fueling Your Body for Energy and Performance

To ensure you're adequately fueling your body for energy and performance, consider implementing the following action steps into your nutrition and hydration routine:

1. Track Your Caloric Intake: Use a food journal or mobile app to track your daily calorie intake and macronutrient distribution. This can help ensure you're meeting your energy needs and maintaining a balanced diet to support your activity level and performance goals.

2. Adjust Portions Based on Activity Level: Tailor your portion sizes and macronutrient ratios

based on your individual energy expenditure and activity level. Consider increasing carbohydrate intake before and after workouts to fuel performance and support recovery.

3. Stay Hydrated: Drink water regularly throughout the day and pay attention to your hydration status, particularly during exercise or in hot weather. Monitor urine color and frequency as indicators of hydration status and aim to consume electrolyte-rich fluids as needed.

4. Plan Balanced Meals and Snacks: Prioritize nutrient-dense, whole foods, including lean proteins, complex carbohydrates, healthy fats, fruits, and vegetables. Plan balanced meals and snacks that provide sustained energy and support recovery and performance.

5. Listen to Your Body: Pay attention to hunger and satiety cues, and honor your body's signals for fueling and hydration. Experiment with different foods, meal timing, and hydration strategies to find what works best for you and supports your energy needs and performance goals.

Conclusion: Fostering Energy and Performance Through Nutrition

In conclusion, fueling your body for energy and performance requires a balanced approach to nutrition and hydration. By understanding the principles of energy balance, optimizing macronutrient ratios, prioritizing pre and post-workout nutrition, debunking myths surrounding fad diets, and emphasizing hydration, you can support your body's energy needs and enhance performance. Implementing actionable steps such as tracking calorie intake, adjusting portions based on activity level, staying hydrated, planning balanced meals and snacks, and listening to your body's signals can help you achieve optimal energy levels and performance outcomes. By prioritizing proper nutrition and hydration, you can unlock your body's full potential and thrive in all aspects of life.

Chapter 05

Hunger Cues and Mindful Eating: Reconnecting with Your Body

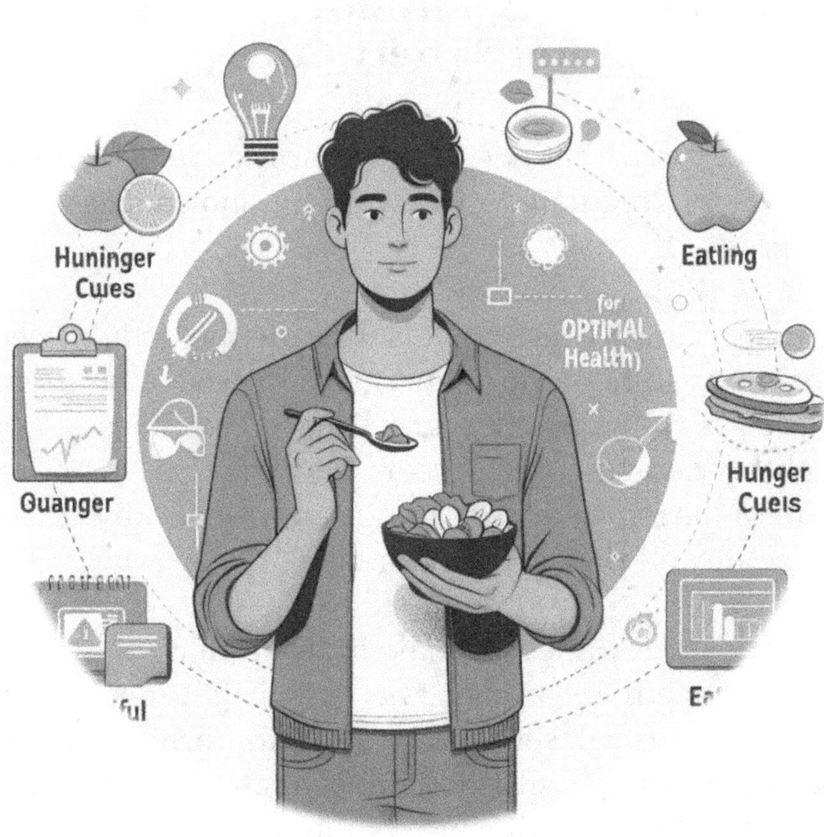

In our fast-paced world filled with distractions and external influences, it's easy to lose touch with our body's natural hunger and satiety cues. This chapter focuses on understanding these physiological signals, embracing mindful eating practices, debunking myths about willpower and deprivation, and nurturing a positive relationship with food for holistic well-being.

Understanding Physiological Hunger and Satiety Cues

Hunger and satiety are complex physiological processes regulated by various hormones and signals in the body.

Hunger Cues: These signals indicate the body's need for nourishment and energy. Physical sensations such as stomach growling, weakness, or lightheadedness may accompany hunger. Ghrelin, often referred to as the "hunger hormone," increases appetite and prompts food intake.

Satiety Cues: Satiety signals indicate that the body's energy needs have been met and it is time to stop eating. Physical sensations such as feeling full or satisfied, along with hormonal signals like leptin, help regulate appetite and food intake.

Embracing Mindful Eating for Healthy Portion Control

Mindful eating is a practice that involves paying attention to the sensory experiences of eating, such as taste, texture, and aroma, as well as internal cues of hunger and satiety. By cultivating awareness and non-judgmental acceptance of food and eating behaviors, mindful eating promotes healthier eating habits and portion control.

Strategies for Mindful Eating:

- Eat Slowly: Take your time to chew each bite thoroughly and savor the flavors and textures of your food.
- Pay Attention: Tune into your body's hunger and satiety signals throughout the meal. Pause periodically to assess your level of fullness.
- Eliminate Distractions: Minimize distractions such as television, phones, or computers during meals to fully focus on the eating experience.
- Practice Gratitude: Cultivate gratitude for the nourishment provided by your food and the effort that went into its preparation.

Strategies to Slow Down and Savor Your Food

Slowing down and savoring your food can enhance the enjoyment of meals and promote mindful eating.

Chew Thoroughly: Chewing each bite thoroughly

not only aids in digestion but also allows you to fully experience the flavors and textures of your food.

Engage Your Senses: Take a moment to appreciate the aroma, appearance, and taste of your food. Notice the colors, smells, and flavors as you eat.

Practice Mindful Breathing: Incorporate mindful breathing exercises before and during meals to help relax the body and focus the mind on the present moment.

Debunking Myths Surrounding Willpower and Deprivation

Myths about willpower and deprivation often perpetuate unhealthy eating habits and negative relationships with food.

Myth: "Willpower is the key to successful dieting."
Fact: Relying solely on willpower to resist cravings and adhere to strict diets is unsustainable in the long term. Instead of relying on sheer willpower, focus on building sustainable habits, making mindful food choices, and cultivating self-compassion.

Myth: "Deprivation is necessary for weight loss."
Fact: Depriving yourself of foods you enjoy can lead to feelings of deprivation, resentment, and ultimately, binge eating. A balanced approach that

includes a variety of foods in moderation is more sustainable and conducive to long-term success.

Importance of a Positive Relationship with Food

Cultivating a positive relationship with food is essential for overall well-being and mental health.

Mindful Eating: By practicing mindfulness and tuning into your body's hunger and satiety cues, you can develop a healthier relationship with food and eating.

Self-Compassion: Be kind to yourself and practice self-compassion when it comes to food choices and eating behaviors. Avoid self-criticism and negative self-talk, and instead focus on nourishing your body with foods that make you feel good.

Enjoyment: Food is meant to be enjoyed, and eating should be a pleasurable experience. Allow yourself to savor your favorite foods in moderation and without guilt.

Action Steps: Cultivating Mindful Eating Practices

To incorporate mindful eating into your daily life, consider the following action steps:

1. Mindful Breathing: Before meals, take a few deep breaths to center yourself and cultivate a sense of mindfulness.

2. Put Down Your Utensils: Between bites, pause and place your utensils down to give yourself a moment to assess your hunger and fullness cues.

3. Savor Each Bite: Take the time to fully experience the flavors, textures, and aromas of your food. Chew slowly and mindfully.

4. Practice Gratitude: Express gratitude for your food and the nourishment it provides. Reflect on the effort that went into growing, preparing, and serving your meal.

5. Listen to Your Body: Tune into your body's hunger and satiety signals throughout the meal. Eat when you're hungry, and stop when you're satisfied.

Conclusion: Nurturing a Positive Relationship with Food

In conclusion, reconnecting with your body's hunger cues and embracing mindful eating practices can foster a healthier relationship with food and eating. By tuning into your body's signals, slowing down, and savoring your food, you can cultivate greater awareness and enjoyment of the eating experience. Debunking myths surrounding willpower and deprivation and emphasizing self-compassion and enjoyment can further support a positive relationship with food. By practicing mindful eating techniques and cultivating a sense of gratitude and self-compassion, you can nourish your body, mind, and soul, fostering overall well-being and vitality.

Part 2:
Building a Healthy and Sustainable Eating Pattern

Chapter 06

Building a Balanced Plate: Putting it all Together

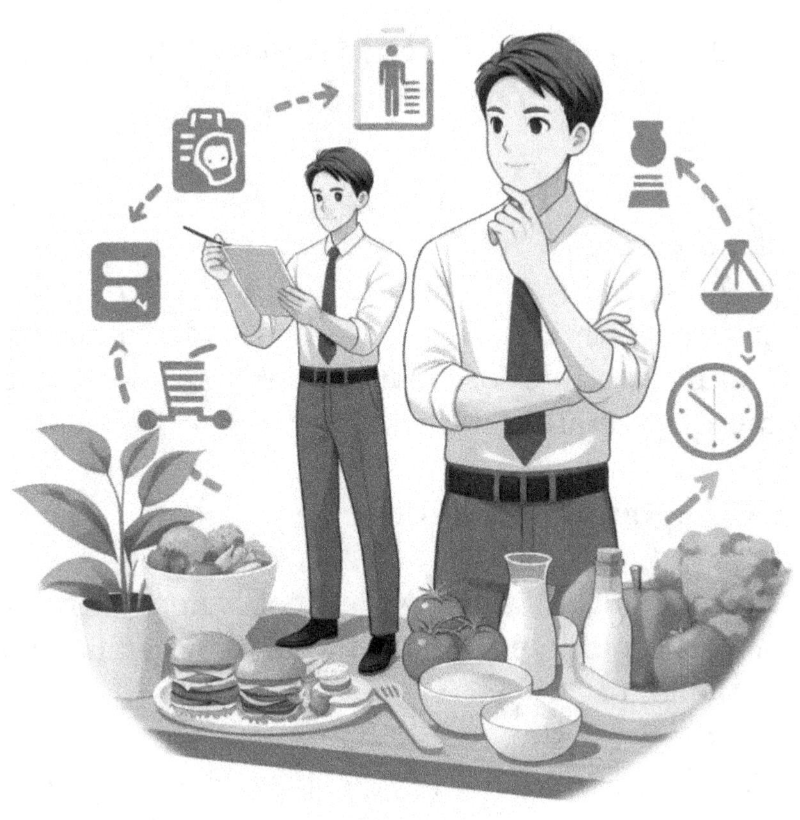

Creating a balanced plate is a cornerstone of healthy eating, ensuring that you provide your body with the nutrients it needs for optimal function and wellbeing. In this chapter, we will explore the concept of MyPlate or similar balanced eating models, discuss strategies for portion control and incorporating all food groups into your diet, debunk myths about demonizing specific food groups, and emphasize the importance of variety and cultural considerations when planning meals.

Understanding MyPlate and Balanced Eating Models

MyPlate is a visual representation of a balanced meal, dividing a plate into sections for fruits, vegetables, grains, and protein, with a side of dairy or dairy alternative. This model provides a simple and intuitive guide for creating balanced meals and promoting overall health and nutrition.

Key Components of MyPlate:

- Fruits: Emphasize a variety of colorful fruits, which provide essential vitamins, minerals, and antioxidants.
- Vegetables: Aim to fill half your plate with a colorful assortment of vegetables, including leafy greens, cruciferous vegetables, and starchy vegetables.
- Grains: Choose whole grains such as brown rice,

quinoa, oats, and whole wheat bread to provide fiber, vitamins, and minerals.

- Protein: Include lean sources of protein such as poultry, fish, beans, lentils, tofu, and nuts to support muscle repair and growth.
- Dairy (or Dairy Alternatives): Incorporate low-fat or non-fat dairy products or fortified dairy alternatives like almond milk or soy milk for calcium and vitamin D.

Creating Balanced Meals with Appropriate Portion Sizes

Balanced meals should consist of a variety of nutrient-rich foods in appropriate portion sizes to meet your energy needs and promote satiety.

Portion Control Tips:

- Use smaller plates and bowls to help control portion sizes and prevent overeating.
- Fill half your plate with vegetables and divide the remaining half between grains and protein.
- Use your hand as a guide for portion sizes: a palm-sized portion of protein, a fist-sized portion of grains, and two cupped handfuls of vegetables.
- Be mindful of calorie-dense foods like oils, nuts, and cheese, and use them sparingly to avoid excessive calorie intake.

Strategies to Incorporate All Food Groups into Your Diet

To ensure you're meeting your nutritional needs, aim to incorporate foods from all food groups into your meals and snacks throughout the day.

Tips for Balancing Food Groups:

- Plan meals around a variety of foods from each food group, including fruits, vegetables, whole grains, lean proteins, and healthy fats.
- Experiment with different cooking methods and flavor combinations to keep meals interesting and enjoyable.
- Get creative with meal prep and batch cooking to streamline the process of incorporating diverse foods into your diet.

Debunking Myths Surrounding Demonizing Specific Food Groups

Myths about demonizing specific food groups can lead to restrictive eating patterns and nutrient deficiencies. It's essential to recognize that all food groups have a place in a balanced diet when consumed in moderation.

Myth: "Carbohydrates are bad for you and should be avoided."

Fact: Carbohydrates are a primary source of energy for the body and are found in nutrient-rich foods like fruits, vegetables, whole grains, and legumes. Choosing whole, minimally processed carbohydrates can provide essential nutrients and fiber for optimal health.

Myth: "Fats make you fat and should be eliminated from your diet."
Fact: Healthy fats, such as those found in avocados, nuts, seeds, olive oil, and fatty fish, are essential for brain health, hormone production, and nutrient absorption. Including moderate amounts of healthy fats in your diet can support overall health and satiety.

Importance of Variety and Cultural Considerations

Variety is essential for ensuring you get a wide range of nutrients and flavors in your diet. Embrace cultural diversity and explore different cuisines to expand your culinary horizons and enjoy a more varied diet.

Cultural Considerations:

- Incorporate traditional foods and recipes from your cultural background into your meal planning.
- Explore cuisines from around the world and

experiment with new ingredients and flavor profiles.
- Be mindful of cultural food traditions and rituals, which can enhance the enjoyment and significance of meals.

Action Steps: Planning Balanced Meals and Snacks

To implement the principles of balanced eating into your daily life, consider the following action steps:

1. Meal Planning: Set aside time each week to plan your meals and snacks, incorporating foods from all food groups.
2. Grocery Shopping: Create a shopping list based on your meal plan and prioritize purchasing a variety of fruits, vegetables, whole grains, lean proteins, and healthy fats.
3. Batch Cooking: Prepare large batches of staple foods like grains, proteins, and vegetables to use in multiple meals throughout the week.
4. Portion Control: Use portion control tools like measuring cups, spoons, and your hand to help visualize appropriate portion sizes.
5. Enjoyment: Focus on enjoying a wide variety of foods and flavors, and embrace cultural diversity in your culinary choices.

Conclusion: Building a Balanced Plate for Optimal Nutrition

In conclusion, building a balanced plate is essential for promoting optimal nutrition and overall health. By following principles like MyPlate, practicing portion control, incorporating foods from all food groups, debunking myths about demonizing specific food groups, and embracing cultural diversity in your diet, you can create meals that nourish your body and satisfy your taste buds. By planning balanced meals and snacks and focusing on enjoyment and variety, you can cultivate a healthy and sustainable eating pattern that supports your long-term health and well-being.

Navigating the Grocery Store: Making Smart Choices

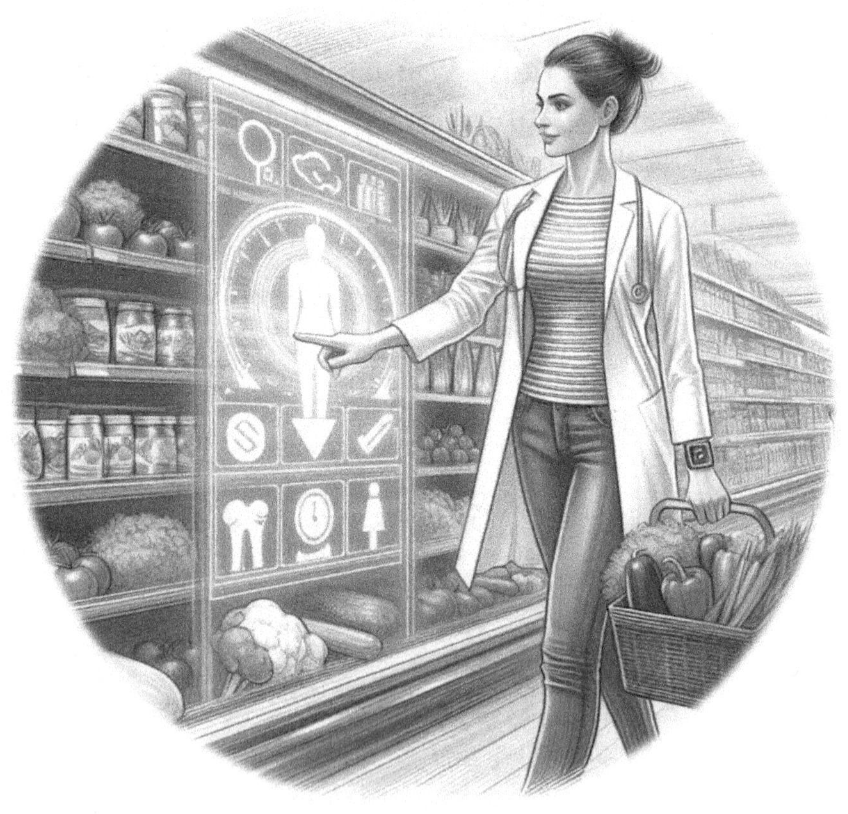

The grocery store can be a maze of options, making it challenging to make healthy choices amidst the abundance of processed foods and marketing gimmicks. In this chapter, we'll explore strategies for deciphering food labels, making healthier swaps, practicing mindful shopping, debunking marketing myths, and implementing actionable steps to navigate the grocery store with confidence and make smart choices for your health.

Strategies for Reading Food Labels and Understanding Ingredients

Understanding how to interpret food labels can empower you to make informed decisions about the products you purchase and consume.

Key Components of Food Labels:

- Ingredients List: Scan the ingredients list to identify any additives, preservatives, or artificial ingredients. Aim for products with simple, recognizable ingredients and avoid those with long lists of additives.
- Nutrition Facts: Pay attention to serving size, calories, and nutrient content per serving. Look for products lower in added sugars, saturated fats, and sodium, and higher in fiber, vitamins, and minerals.
- Allergen Information: Check for allergen warnings if you have food allergies or

sensitivities to avoid potential adverse reactions.

Exploring Healthy Swaps for Processed Foods

Making healthier swaps for processed foods can help reduce your intake of added sugars, unhealthy fats, and artificial ingredients while increasing your consumption of nutrient-dense whole foods.

Healthy Swaps to Consider:

- Whole Grains: Choose whole grain options like brown rice, quinoa, whole wheat bread, and oats instead of refined grains like white rice and white bread.

- Fresh Produce: Opt for fresh fruits and vegetables over canned or processed varieties whenever possible to maximize nutrient content and flavor.

- Lean Proteins: Select lean sources of protein such as poultry, fish, tofu, beans, and legumes instead of processed meats like deli meats and sausages.

- Healthy Fats: Incorporate sources of healthy fats like avocados, nuts, seeds, and olive oil in place of trans fats and hydrogenated oils found in many processed foods.

Highlighting the Importance of Mindful Shopping

Practicing mindful shopping involves being intentional and aware of your food choices, avoiding impulsive purchases, and prioritizing whole, nutrient-dense foods.

Mindful Shopping Tips:

- Plan Ahead: Create a grocery list based on your meal plan and nutritional needs to avoid wandering aimlessly and making impulse purchases.
- Shop the Perimeter: Focus on shopping the perimeter of the grocery store, where fresh produce, lean proteins, dairy, and whole grains are typically located.
- Read Labels Carefully: Take the time to read food labels and ingredient lists, and be wary of misleading marketing claims that may exaggerate the healthfulness of a product.
- Stick to Your Budget: Set a budget for your grocery trip and stick to it by prioritizing essentials and avoiding unnecessary purchases.

Debunking Myths Surrounding Marketing Claims and "Healthy" Labeling

Food labels and marketing claims can be misleading, making it essential to look beyond buzzwords and marketing hype to make truly informed choices.

Myth: "Natural means healthy."
Fact: The term "natural" is not regulated by the FDA and can be used arbitrarily by food manufacturers. A product labeled as "natural" may still contain artificial additives, preservatives, or high levels of added sugars or sodium.

Myth: "Low-fat or fat-free is always healthier."
Fact: Many low-fat or fat-free products compensate for the reduced fat content by adding extra sugar, salt, or artificial additives to enhance flavor. In some cases, opting for the full-fat version may be a better choice, especially if it contains healthy fats and fewer processed ingredients.

Action Steps: Making Smart Choices at the Grocery Store

To make smart choices at the grocery store, consider implementing the following action steps:

1. Plan Your Grocery List: Before heading to the

store, create a detailed grocery list based on your meal plan and nutritional needs.

2. Prioritize Whole Foods: Focus on purchasing whole, minimally processed foods like fruits, vegetables, lean proteins, whole grains, and healthy fats.

3. Read Labels Thoroughly: Take the time to read food labels and ingredient lists carefully, paying attention to serving sizes, nutrient content, and added sugars, fats, and sodium.

4. Avoid Impulse Buys: Stick to your grocery list and avoid making impulsive purchases by staying focused on your nutritional goals and budget.

5. Shop Mindfully: Practice mindfulness while shopping, remaining aware of marketing tactics and choosing products that align with your values and health priorities.

Conclusion: Navigating the Grocery Store with Confidence

In conclusion, navigating the grocery store can be a daunting task, but with the right strategies and mindset, you can make smart choices that support your health and well-being. By understanding how to read food labels, making healthier swaps for processed foods, practicing mindful shopping, and debunking myths surrounding marketing claims, you can shop with confidence and make informed decisions about the foods you bring into your home.

By prioritizing whole, nutrient-dense foods and avoiding impulse purchases, you can create a pantry stocked with ingredients that nourish your body and support your long-term health goals.

Chapter 08

Eating on the Go and Dining Out: Maintaining Healthy Habits

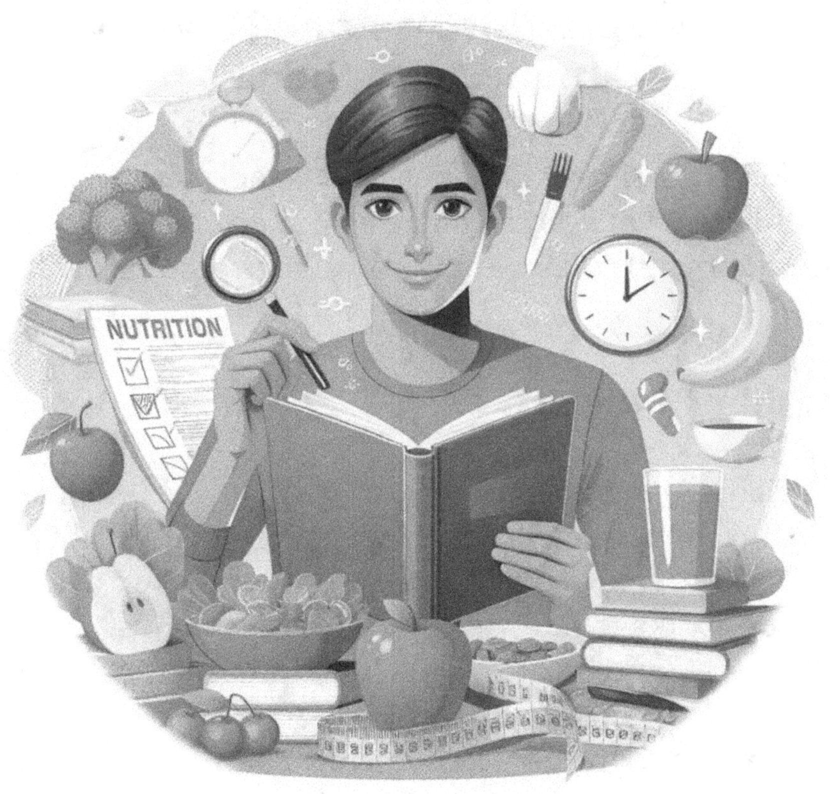

Maintaining healthy eating habits can be challenging when faced with busy schedules and dining out temptations. In this chapter, we'll explore strategies for packing nutritious meals and snacks for busy days, tips for making healthier choices when dining out, the importance of portion control and mindful eating, debunking myths about skipping meals or opting for fast food, and actionable steps to help you maintain healthy habits while on the go.

Strategies for Packing Healthy Lunches and Snacks

Packing nutritious lunches and snacks is essential for fueling your body and sustaining energy levels throughout the day, especially when you're on the go.

Healthy Packing Tips:

- Plan Ahead: Dedicate time each week to plan and prepare meals and snacks for the days ahead.
- Choose Nutrient-Dense Foods: Opt for whole foods like fruits, vegetables, lean proteins, whole grains, and healthy fats that provide sustained energy and essential nutrients.
- Portion Control: Use portion control containers or resealable bags to pack appropriate serving sizes and avoid overeating.
- Include Variety: Mix and match different food groups to ensure a balance of flavors, textures,

and nutrients in your meals and snacks.

Tips for Making Healthy Choices When Dining Out

Eating out at restaurants can present challenges to maintaining healthy habits, but with a few mindful strategies, you can make nutritious choices that align with your health goals.

Healthy Dining Out Tips:

- Review the Menu Ahead of Time: Take a look at the menu online beforehand to identify healthier options and plan your meal in advance.
- Choose Wisely: Opt for grilled or baked proteins, steamed vegetables, whole grains, and salads with dressing on the side instead of fried or heavily sauced dishes.
- Ask for Modifications: Don't hesitate to ask for substitutions or modifications to accommodate your dietary preferences or restrictions, such as swapping fries for a side salad or requesting sauces on the side.
- Practice Portion Control: Be mindful of portion sizes, and consider sharing entrees or taking half of your meal home for later.

Importance of Portion Control and Mindful Eating

Portion control and mindful eating are essential practices for maintaining a healthy relationship with food and preventing overeating, especially when dining out or on the go.

Portion Control Tips:

- Use Visual Cues: Estimate portion sizes using visual cues, such as comparing servings to familiar objects like a deck of cards (protein), tennis ball (fruit), or fist (grains).
- Listen to Your Body: Pay attention to hunger and satiety cues, and stop eating when you feel satisfied rather than overly full.
- Slow Down: Take your time to chew your food thoroughly, savor the flavors, and enjoy the dining experience.

Debunking Myths Surrounding Skipping Meals or Fast Food Options

Myths about skipping meals or relying on fast food for convenience can sabotage your efforts to maintain a healthy diet and lifestyle.

Myth: "Skipping meals is an effective way to lose weight."

Fact: Skipping meals can disrupt your metabolism, lead to overeating later in the day, and cause fluctuations in energy levels and mood. Instead of skipping meals, focus on eating balanced meals and snacks throughout the day to support sustained energy and satiety.

Myth: "Fast food is the only option when you're on the go."
Fact: While fast food may be convenient, it often lacks the nutritional quality of homemade or freshly prepared meals. With proper planning and preparation, you can pack nutritious meals and snacks to enjoy on the go without resorting to fast food options.

Action Steps: Preparing Grab-and-Go Snacks for Busy Schedules

To incorporate healthy eating habits into your busy lifestyle, consider the following action steps:

1. Stock Up on Portable Snacks: Keep a supply of grab-and-go snacks like fruits, nuts, seeds, yogurt, hummus, and whole grain crackers on hand for quick and convenient options when you're on the go.
2. Prep Ahead: Dedicate time each week to prepare and portion out snacks in advance, making it easier to grab nutritious options when you're in a hurry.

3. Invest in Portable Containers: Invest in reusable containers or snack bags to pack your snacks for easy transport and portion control.
4. Stay Hydrated: Don't forget to pack water or other hydrating beverages to stay hydrated throughout the day and prevent mistaking thirst for hunger.
5. Listen to Your Body: Pay attention to your body's hunger and satiety cues, and honor your hunger with nourishing snacks when needed.

Conclusion: Maintaining Healthy Habits On the Go and While Dining Out

In conclusion, maintaining healthy eating habits while on the go and dining out requires planning, mindfulness, and flexibility. By packing nutritious meals and snacks, making smart choices when dining out, practicing portion control and mindful eating, and debunking myths about skipping meals or resorting to fast food, you can prioritize your health and well-being no matter where life takes you. By incorporating actionable steps like preparing grab-and-go snacks and listening to your body's cues, you can stay on track with your health goals and enjoy a balanced and fulfilling lifestyle.

Chapter 09

Hydration: The Unsung Hero of Health

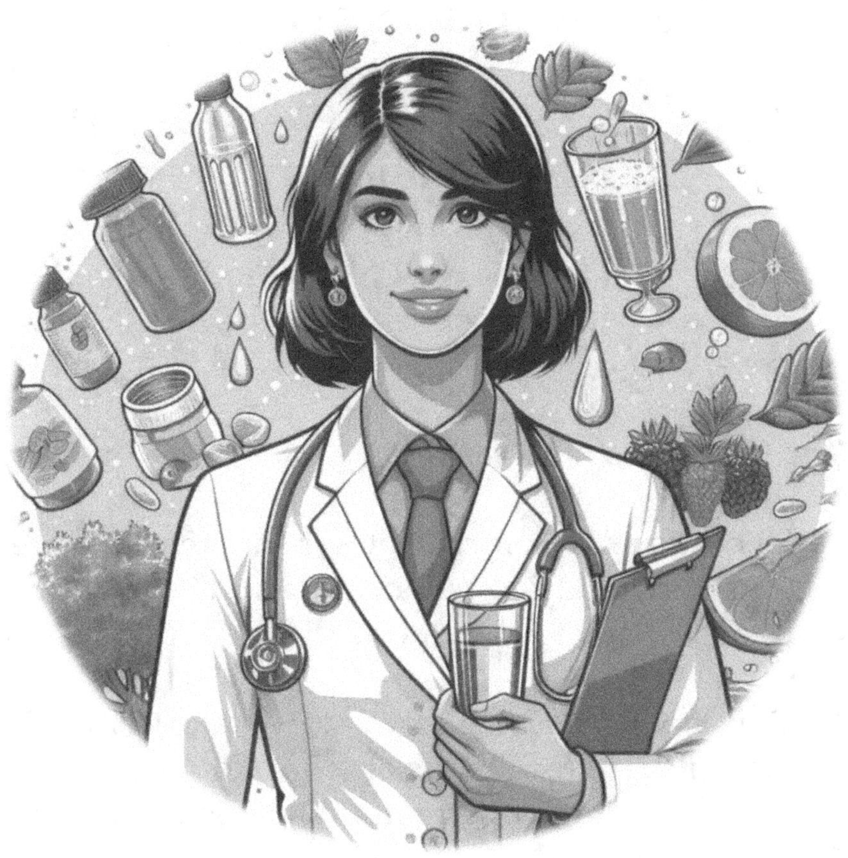

Water is often overlooked, yet it plays a crucial role in maintaining overall health and well-being. In this chapter, we'll dive into the importance of water for various bodily functions, explore factors influencing individual hydration needs, discuss the benefits of staying hydrated, debunk myths surrounding alternatives to water, highlight strategies for increasing water intake, and provide actionable steps to prioritize hydration in your daily life.

Importance of Water for Various Bodily Functions

Water is essential for nearly every bodily function, serving as a vital component of cells, tissues, and organs.

Key Functions of Water:

- Hydration: Water regulates body temperature, transports nutrients and oxygen to cells, and removes waste products through urine and sweat.
- Digestion: Adequate water intake aids in digestion by facilitating the breakdown of food and absorption of nutrients in the digestive tract.
- Cognitive Function: Staying hydrated supports optimal brain function, improving focus, concentration, and cognitive performance.
- Joint Health: Water lubricates joints and cushions tissues, reducing friction and supporting joint

mobility and flexibility.

Factors Influencing Individual Hydration Needs

Individual hydration needs vary based on factors such as age, body size, activity level, climate, and overall health status.

Factors Affecting Hydration Needs:

- Activity Level: Active individuals and those engaging in strenuous exercise require more water to compensate for fluid loss through sweating.
- Climate: Hot and humid environments increase sweat production and evaporative water loss, necessitating higher fluid intake.
- Medical Conditions: Certain medical conditions such as fever, diarrhea, and kidney disease can increase fluid requirements and the risk of dehydration.
- Pregnancy and Lactation: Pregnant and breastfeeding women have increased fluid needs to support fetal development, milk production, and hydration.

Benefits of Staying Hydrated

Maintaining adequate hydration offers numerous

health benefits, including improved energy levels, digestion, and cognitive function.

Benefits of Hydration:

- Energy Levels: Proper hydration helps maintain optimal energy levels and reduces feelings of fatigue and lethargy.
- Digestive Health: Water aids in digestion by softening stools and facilitating the movement of food through the digestive tract, preventing constipation and promoting regularity.
- Cognitive Function: Staying hydrated supports cognitive function, memory, and concentration, enhancing overall mental clarity and performance.
- Physical Performance: Adequate hydration improves athletic performance, endurance, and recovery by regulating body temperature and reducing the risk of dehydration-related fatigue and cramping.

Debunking Myths Surrounding Sugary Drinks and Detoxes

While sugary drinks and detoxes may claim to hydrate the body, they often fall short of providing the same benefits as water and may even have detrimental effects on health.

Myth: "Sugary Drinks Hydrate You as Well as

Water."

Fact: Sugary drinks like soda, fruit juices, and energy drinks may provide fluid, but they also contain added sugars, which can contribute to weight gain, tooth decay, and chronic health conditions like diabetes and heart disease. Water remains the best choice for hydration without the added sugars and empty calories.

Myth: "Detoxes and Cleanses are Superior to Water for Hydration."

Fact: Detoxes and cleanses often involve restrictive diets or liquid-only regimens, which may lead to dehydration and nutrient deficiencies. While some detox beverages may contain hydrating ingredients like water or herbal teas, they lack the balance of nutrients provided by whole foods and can be unsustainable and potentially harmful in the long term.

Strategies for Incorporating Water Throughout the Day

Increasing water intake can be achieved through simple strategies and habits that promote hydration.

Tips for Increasing Water Intake:

- Carry a Reusable Water Bottle: Keep a reusable water bottle with you throughout the day as a reminder to drink water regularly.

- Set Reminders: Use smartphone apps or alarms to set reminders to drink water at regular intervals, especially if you tend to forget.
- Flavor Infusions: Enhance the flavor of water with natural additions like fresh fruits, herbs, or cucumber slices to make it more enticing and enjoyable.
- Eat Hydrating Foods: Incorporate hydrating foods with high water content, such as fruits (e.g., watermelon, oranges), vegetables (e.g., cucumbers, celery), and soups, into your meals and snacks.
- Monitor Urine Color: Use urine color as a simple indicator of hydration status; aim for pale yellow urine as a sign of adequate hydration.

Action Steps: Prioritizing Hydration in Your Daily Life

To prioritize hydration in your daily life, consider implementing the following action steps:

1. Carry a Reusable Water Bottle: Invest in a durable, BPA-free water bottle and carry it with you wherever you go to ensure easy access to hydration.
2. Set Hydration Goals: Establish daily hydration goals based on your individual needs and lifestyle factors, aiming for a specific volume of water intake per day.
3. Track Your Intake: Use a hydration tracking app

or journal to monitor your daily water intake and progress toward your hydration goals.

4. Incorporate Hydration Breaks: Schedule regular hydration breaks throughout the day, such as during transitions between activities or at designated times during work or school.

5. Lead by Example: Encourage family members, friends, and colleagues to prioritize hydration by modeling healthy hydration habits and sharing the benefits of staying hydrated.

Conclusion: Embracing Water as the Unsung Hero of Health

In conclusion, water serves as the unsung hero of health, playing a vital role in supporting various bodily functions and promoting overall well-being. By understanding the importance of hydration, recognizing individual hydration needs, embracing the benefits of staying hydrated, debunking myths surrounding sugary drinks and detoxes, and implementing strategies for increasing water intake, you can prioritize hydration in your daily life and reap the rewards of improved energy, digestion, and cognitive function. By carrying a reusable water bottle, setting reminders to drink water, and incorporating hydrating foods and beverages into your diet, you can ensure that water remains a cornerstone of your health and wellness routine.

Chapter 10

Building a Sustainable Eating Pattern for Life

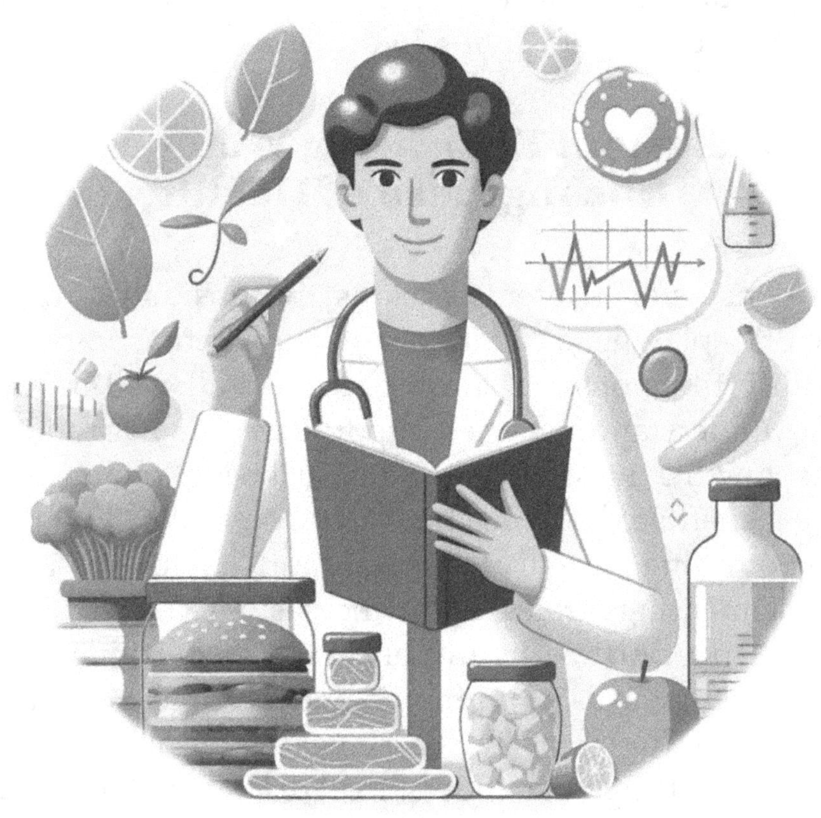

Creating a sustainable eating pattern is not just about following a set of rules; it's about developing a positive and flexible relationship with food that supports your long-term health and well-being. In this final chapter, we'll delve into the concept of intuitive eating and body awareness, explore strategies for fostering a healthy relationship with food, highlight the importance of balance and flexibility, debunk myths surrounding perfectionism and guilt, emphasize the value of sustainable habits, and provide actionable steps to cultivate a sustainable eating pattern that lasts a lifetime.

Understanding Intuitive Eating and Body Awareness

Intuitive eating is a holistic approach to nourishing your body, focusing on listening to your body's cues, honoring your hunger and fullness, and embracing food without judgment.

Key Principles of Intuitive Eating:

- Reject the Diet Mentality: Let go of restrictive dieting and embrace a non-diet approach that prioritizes satisfaction and well-being over weight loss.
- Honor Your Hunger: Learn to recognize and respond to your body's hunger signals by eating when you're hungry and stopping when you're

comfortably full.

- Respect Your Fullness: Listen to your body's cues of fullness and satisfaction, and stop eating when you feel satisfied rather than overly full.

- Challenge Food Rules: Challenge rigid food rules and beliefs about "good" and "bad" foods, allowing yourself to enjoy a wide variety of foods without guilt or shame.

- Discover Satisfaction: Cultivate a sense of pleasure and satisfaction in eating by savoring your food, exploring different flavors and textures, and tuning into your taste preferences.

Strategies for Developing a Healthy Relationship with Food

Fostering a healthy relationship with food involves cultivating self-awareness, practicing mindfulness, and embracing balance and moderation in your eating patterns.

Strategies for Food Freedom:

- Practice Mindful Eating: Slow down and pay attention to your eating experience, savoring the flavors, textures, and aromas of your food.

- Cultivate Gratitude: Express gratitude for the nourishment and pleasure that food provides, fostering a positive and appreciative attitude toward eating.

- Embrace Variety: Enjoy a diverse range of foods from all food groups, incorporating different flavors, colors, and cuisines into your meals and snacks.

- Practice Self-Compassion: Be kind and gentle with yourself, letting go of self-criticism and guilt around food choices, and treating yourself with the same kindness and understanding you would offer to a friend.

Importance of Flexibility and Balance in Your Eating Pattern

Flexibility and balance are essential components of a sustainable eating pattern, allowing for enjoyment and satisfaction while also supporting health and well-being.

Benefits of Flexibility and Balance:

- Reduced Stress: Avoiding rigid food rules and restrictions reduces stress and anxiety around eating, promoting a more relaxed and enjoyable relationship with food.

- Improved Mental Health: Embracing flexibility and balance in your eating pattern reduces the risk of disordered eating behaviors and promotes positive body image and self-esteem.

- Enhanced Satisfaction: Allowing yourself to enjoy a wide variety of foods without guilt or deprivation increases satisfaction and pleasure in eating, leading to a more fulfilling and sustainable approach to nutrition.

Debunking Myths Surrounding Perfectionism and Guilt

Perfectionism and guilt surrounding food choices can undermine efforts to maintain a healthy and balanced eating pattern, leading to stress, anxiety, and dissatisfaction.

Myth: "I Have to Eat Perfectly to Be Healthy."
Fact: There is no such thing as perfect eating, and striving for perfection only sets unrealistic expectations and fosters feelings of guilt and inadequacy. Embrace imperfection and focus on progress, not perfection, in your journey toward health and well-being.

Myth: "Indulging Occasionally Means I've Failed."
Fact: Enjoying occasional indulgences is a normal and healthy part of eating, and it's important to let go of guilt and judgment around food choices. Remember that one meal or snack does not define your overall eating pattern, and it's the consistency of your habits over time that matters most.

Emphasizing the Importance of Long-Term Sustainable Habits

Building a sustainable eating pattern is not about quick fixes or short-term solutions; it's about adopting habits that promote health and well-being for life.

Keys to Sustainability:

- Consistency: Focus on making small, gradual changes to your eating habits that you can maintain over the long term, rather than seeking drastic or unsustainable solutions.
- Flexibility: Embrace flexibility and adaptability in your eating patterns, allowing for changes in circumstances, preferences, and goals without derailing your progress.
- Mindfulness: Practice mindfulness and self-awareness in your eating habits, tuning into your body's cues and making choices that align with your values and goals.
- Self-Compassion: Treat yourself with kindness and compassion, acknowledging that setbacks and challenges are a natural part of the journey and learning from them rather than dwelling on them.

Action Steps: Practicing Self-Compassion and Enjoying Food Without Guilt

To cultivate a sustainable eating pattern for life, consider implementing the following action steps:

1. Practice Self-Compassion: Be gentle and understanding with yourself, letting go of perfectionism and embracing imperfection in your eating habits.
2. Challenge Food Guilt: Recognize and challenge feelings of guilt or shame around food choices, reminding yourself that all foods can fit into a balanced and healthy eating pattern.
3. Enjoy Food Mindfully: Savor the experience of eating, paying attention to the flavors, textures, and sensations of each bite, and cultivating gratitude for the nourishment and pleasure that food provides.
4. Let Go of Food Rules: Release rigid food rules and restrictions, allowing yourself to enjoy a wide variety of foods without judgment or deprivation.
5. Focus on Long-Term Habits: Shift your focus from short-term outcomes to long-term habits, prioritizing consistency, flexibility, and self-care in your approach to nutrition and health.

Conclusion: Embracing Sustainable Eating Habits for Life

In conclusion, building a sustainable eating pattern for life is not about following strict rules or achieving perfection; it's about fostering a positive and balanced relationship with food that supports your health and well-being in the long term. By embracing intuitive eating principles, developing a healthy relationship with food, prioritizing flexibility and balance, debunking myths surrounding perfectionism and guilt, and emphasizing the importance of sustainable habits, you can create an eating pattern that nourishes your body, mind, and soul for life. By practicing self-compassion, letting go of food guilt, enjoying food mindfully, and focusing on long-term habits, you can cultivate a sustainable approach to nutrition that promotes health, happiness, and vitality for years to come.

Part 3:
Optimizing Your Health and Wellbeing

Chapter 11

Nutrition and Chronic Disease Prevention

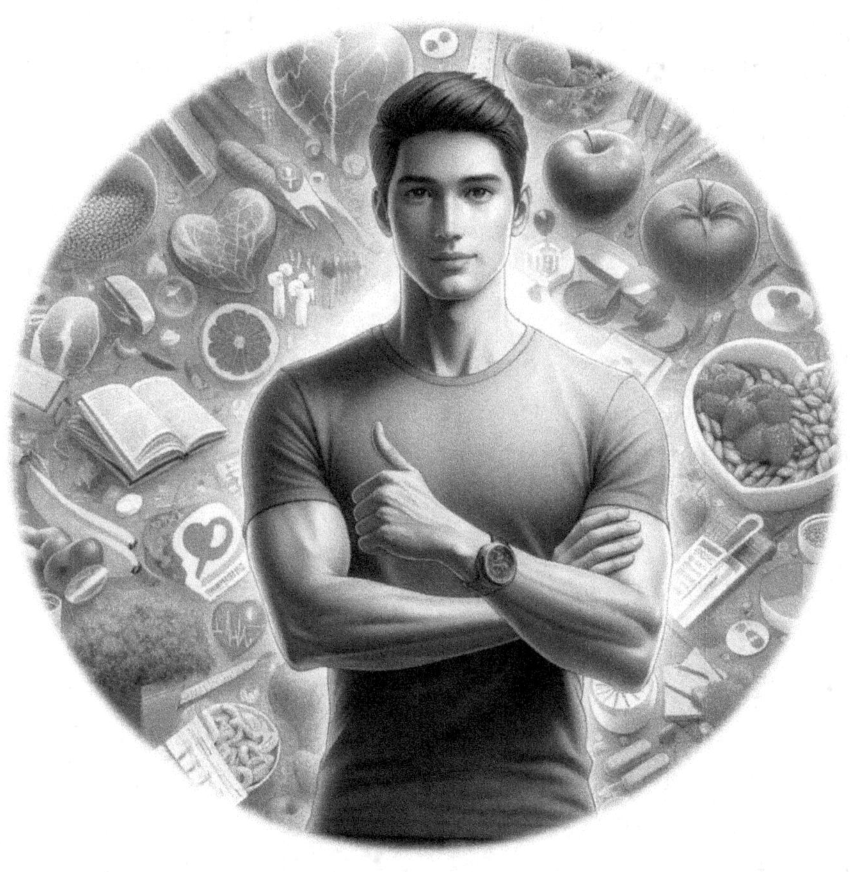

Nutrition plays a pivotal role in preventing chronic diseases such as heart disease, diabetes, and certain cancers. In this chapter, we will delve into the significance of diet in chronic disease prevention, explore the benefits of specific dietary patterns, emphasize the importance of seeking personalized guidance from healthcare professionals, debunk myths surrounding miracle cures and fad diets, and provide actionable steps to integrate anti-inflammatory and nutrient-rich foods into your diet to optimize health and well-being.

The Role of Diet in Chronic Disease Prevention

Dietary choices can significantly impact the development and progression of chronic diseases, making nutrition a powerful tool for prevention and management.

Key Factors in Disease Prevention:

- Heart Disease: A diet rich in fruits, vegetables, whole grains, lean proteins, and healthy fats can help lower cholesterol levels, reduce blood pressure, and decrease the risk of heart disease.
- Diabetes: Consuming a balanced diet that regulates blood sugar levels through controlled carbohydrate intake, fiber-rich foods, and healthy fats can prevent or manage type 2

diabetes.

- Cancer: Certain dietary patterns, such as those high in fruits, vegetables, and antioxidants, may reduce the risk of certain types of cancer by protecting cells from damage and supporting immune function.

Benefits of Specific Dietary Patterns for Health Conditions

Various dietary patterns, such as the Mediterranean diet, DASH diet, and plant-based diets, have been associated with numerous health benefits and may help prevent or manage chronic diseases.

Examples of Beneficial Dietary Patterns:

- Mediterranean Diet: Rich in fruits, vegetables, whole grains, fish, nuts, and olive oil, the Mediterranean diet has been linked to reduced risk of heart disease, stroke, and certain cancers.

- DASH Diet: The Dietary Approaches to Stop Hypertension (DASH) diet emphasizes fruits, vegetables, whole grains, lean proteins, and low-fat dairy products, helping to lower blood pressure and reduce the risk of heart disease.

- Plant-Based Diet: Plant-based diets centered around fruits, vegetables, legumes, nuts, and seeds can lower cholesterol, improve blood sugar control, and reduce the risk of obesity-related conditions.

Importance of Consulting Healthcare Professionals for Guidance

While dietary changes can play a significant role in disease prevention, it's essential to seek personalized guidance from healthcare professionals, such as registered dietitians or physicians, to ensure safe and effective strategies.

Reasons to Consult a Healthcare Professional:

- Personalized Recommendations: Healthcare professionals can provide tailored dietary recommendations based on individual health status, medical history, and dietary preferences.
- Monitoring and Support: Regular monitoring and support from healthcare professionals can help track progress, make adjustments to treatment plans, and address any concerns or challenges that arise.
- Preventing Nutrient Deficiencies: Healthcare professionals can help prevent nutrient deficiencies or imbalances that may occur with certain dietary interventions, ensuring overall nutritional adequacy.

Debunking Myths Surrounding Miracle Cures and Fad Diets

It's essential to be wary of miracle cures and fad diets that promise quick fixes for chronic diseases, as they may lack scientific evidence and could potentially be harmful.

Myth: "A Single Food or Supplement Can Cure Chronic Diseases."

Fact: While certain foods and nutrients may offer health benefits, there is no single miracle cure for chronic diseases. Instead, focus on adopting a balanced and varied diet that includes a wide range of nutrient-rich foods to support overall health and well-being.

Myth: "Fad Diets Provide Long-Term Solutions for Disease Prevention."

Fact: Fad diets often promote restrictive eating patterns that are unsustainable and may lead to nutrient deficiencies, disordered eating behaviors, and long-term health consequences. Instead of following fads, prioritize evidence-based dietary recommendations supported by scientific research.

Action Steps: Incorporating Anti-Inflammatory and Nutrient-Rich Foods

To optimize health and well-being and reduce the risk of chronic diseases, consider implementing the following action steps:

1. Focus on Whole Foods: Incorporate a variety of whole, minimally processed foods into your diet, including fruits, vegetables, whole grains, lean proteins, and healthy fats.
2. Prioritize Anti-Inflammatory Foods: Include foods rich in anti-inflammatory nutrients, such as omega-3 fatty acids (found in fatty fish, flaxseeds, and walnuts), antioxidants (found in colorful fruits and vegetables), and spices (such as turmeric and ginger).
3. Limit Processed Foods: Reduce consumption of processed and ultra-processed foods high in added sugars, unhealthy fats, and sodium, which can contribute to inflammation and chronic disease risk.
4. Stay Hydrated: Drink plenty of water throughout the day to support hydration and overall health, as adequate hydration is essential for cellular function and disease prevention.
5. Seek Professional Guidance: Consult with a registered dietitian or healthcare provider to develop a personalized nutrition plan tailored to your individual needs, goals, and health status.

Conclusion: Empowering Health Through Nutrition and Lifestyle

In conclusion, nutrition plays a fundamental role in preventing chronic diseases and promoting optimal health and well-being. By adopting a balanced diet rich in anti-inflammatory and nutrient-rich foods, seeking personalized guidance from healthcare professionals, and debunking myths surrounding miracle cures and fad diets, you can empower yourself to take control of your health and reduce the risk of chronic diseases. By incorporating actionable steps to integrate healthy eating habits into your lifestyle, you can cultivate a foundation of wellness that supports lifelong health and vitality. Remember that small changes can lead to significant improvements in health over time, and prioritizing self-care and preventive strategies is key to achieving lasting well-being.

Chapter 12

Nutrition and Mental Health

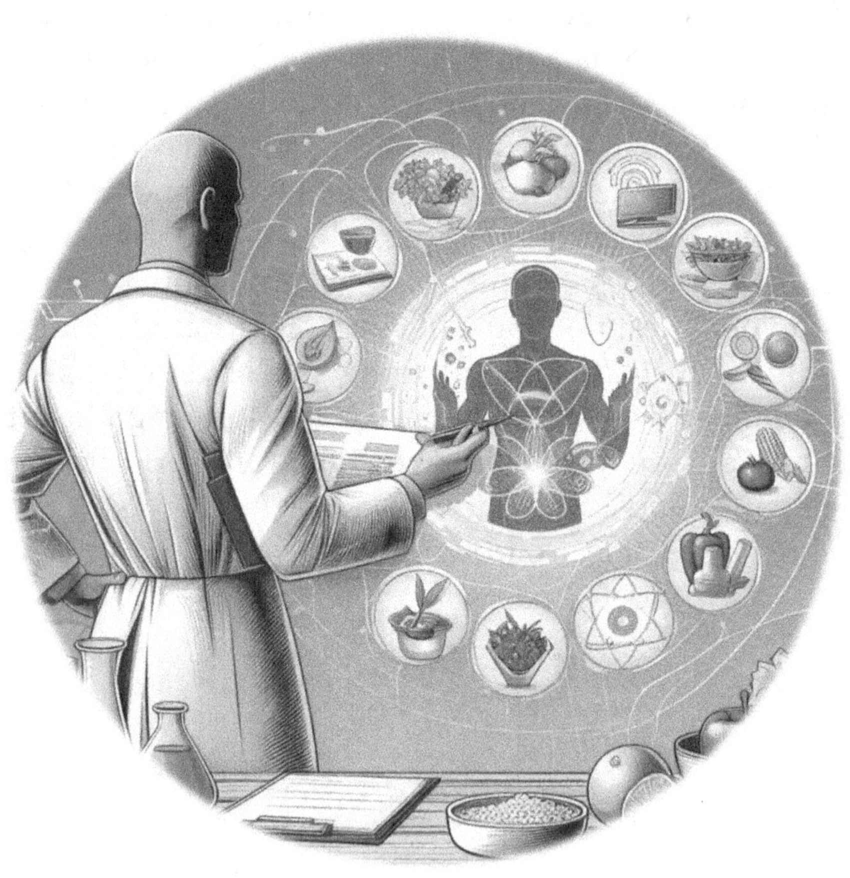

The connection between nutrition and mental health is profound, with emerging research highlighting the intricate interplay between gut health, diet, and overall well-being. In this chapter, we'll delve into the link between gut health, explore the role of specific nutrients in supporting mood and cognitive function, emphasize the importance of managing stress and sleep, debunk myths surrounding miracle cures for mental health conditions, and provide actionable steps to prioritize a balanced diet and healthy lifestyle practices for optimal mental well-being.

The Gut-Brain Connection: Exploring the Link Between Gut Health and Mental Well-being

The gut-brain axis, a bidirectional communication system between the gut and the brain, plays a crucial role in regulating mood, emotions, and cognitive function.

Key Aspects of the Gut-Brain Connection:

- Microbiota Composition: The balance of bacteria in the gut, known as the microbiota, influences neurotransmitter production, inflammation, and stress response, impacting mental health.
- Neurotransmitter Production: Gut bacteria produce neurotransmitters like serotonin and dopamine, which play key roles in mood

regulation and emotional well-being.

- Immune System Regulation: The gut microbiota modulates immune function and inflammation, which can impact mental health conditions such as depression and anxiety.

Role of Specific Nutrients in Supporting Mood and Cognitive Function

Certain nutrients play essential roles in brain health and mental well-being, supporting neurotransmitter synthesis, neural connectivity, and cognitive function.

Nutrients for Mental Health:

- Omega-3 Fatty Acids: Found in fatty fish, flaxseeds, and walnuts, omega-3 fatty acids support brain structure and function, reducing inflammation and supporting mood regulation.
- B Vitamins: B vitamins, including folate, vitamin B12, and vitamin B6, are involved in neurotransmitter synthesis and methylation, contributing to mood stability and cognitive function.
- Antioxidants: Antioxidants such as vitamin C, vitamin E, and flavonoids protect brain cells from oxidative stress and inflammation, supporting cognitive function and mood regulation.

Importance of Managing Stress and Sleep for Optimal Mental Health

Stress management and adequate sleep are critical components of mental well-being, influencing mood, cognition, and overall quality of life.

Stress Management Strategies:

- Mindfulness and Meditation: Practices like mindfulness meditation, deep breathing exercises, and progressive muscle relaxation can reduce stress levels and promote emotional balance.
- Physical Activity: Regular exercise releases endorphins, reduces cortisol levels, and improves mood, serving as a powerful stress-relief strategy.
- Social Support: Building strong social connections and seeking support from friends, family, or support groups can buffer the effects of stress and promote resilience.

Sleep Hygiene Practices:

- Consistent Sleep Schedule: Maintain a consistent sleep schedule, going to bed and waking up at the same time each day to regulate your body's internal clock.
- Create a Restful Environment: Create a sleep-

friendly environment by minimizing noise, light, and electronic devices in the bedroom, and ensuring your mattress and pillows provide adequate comfort and support.

- Limit Stimulants Before Bed: Avoid caffeine, nicotine, and alcohol close to bedtime, as they can disrupt sleep patterns and impair sleep quality.

Debunking Myths Surrounding Specific Foods or Supplements for Mental Health Conditions

While certain foods and nutrients can support mental well-being, it's essential to debunk myths surrounding miracle cures or quick fixes for mental health conditions.

Myth: "A Specific Food or Supplement Can Cure Depression."
Fact: While nutrition plays a role in mental health, there is no single food or supplement that can cure depression or other mental health conditions. Instead, focus on adopting a balanced diet and lifestyle that supports overall well-being.

Myth: "Herbal Supplements Are Safer and More Effective Than Prescription Medications."
Fact: Herbal supplements may have potential benefits for mental health, but they can also interact with medications and may not be regulated or

standardized for quality and safety. It's essential to consult with a healthcare professional before using herbal supplements for mental health concerns.

Action Steps: Prioritizing a Balanced Diet and Healthy Lifestyle Practices for Mental Well-being

To prioritize mental well-being and support optimal brain health, consider implementing the following action steps:

1. Eat a Balanced Diet: Focus on consuming a varied and nutrient-rich diet that includes fruits, vegetables, whole grains, lean proteins, and healthy fats to support brain health and mood regulation.
2. Manage Stress: Incorporate stress-reduction techniques such as mindfulness, meditation, and physical activity into your daily routine to promote emotional resilience and well-being.
3. Prioritize Sleep: Establish a regular sleep schedule, create a restful sleep environment, and practice good sleep hygiene habits to ensure restorative and restful sleep each night.
4. Seek Professional Help: If you're struggling with mental health concerns, don't hesitate to reach out to a qualified mental health professional for support, guidance, and treatment options tailored to your individual needs.
5. Stay Informed: Stay informed about the latest

research and evidence-based recommendations for mental health and nutrition, and be wary of misinformation or unfounded claims about miracle cures or quick fixes.

Conclusion: Nourishing the Mind-Body Connection for Optimal Mental Well-being

In conclusion, nutrition plays a pivotal role in supporting mental health and well-being, with the gut-brain connection serving as a powerful link between diet and mental well-being. By prioritizing gut health, incorporating nutrient-rich foods into your diet, managing stress, and prioritizing sleep, you can optimize brain function, mood regulation, and overall mental well-being. Remember to debunk myths surrounding miracle cures and quick fixes, and instead focus on adopting a balanced diet and healthy lifestyle practices that support long-term mental health and resilience. By taking proactive steps to nourish the mind-body connection, you can cultivate emotional balance, resilience, and vitality, allowing you to thrive in all aspects of life.

Chapter 13

Nutrition and Weight Management

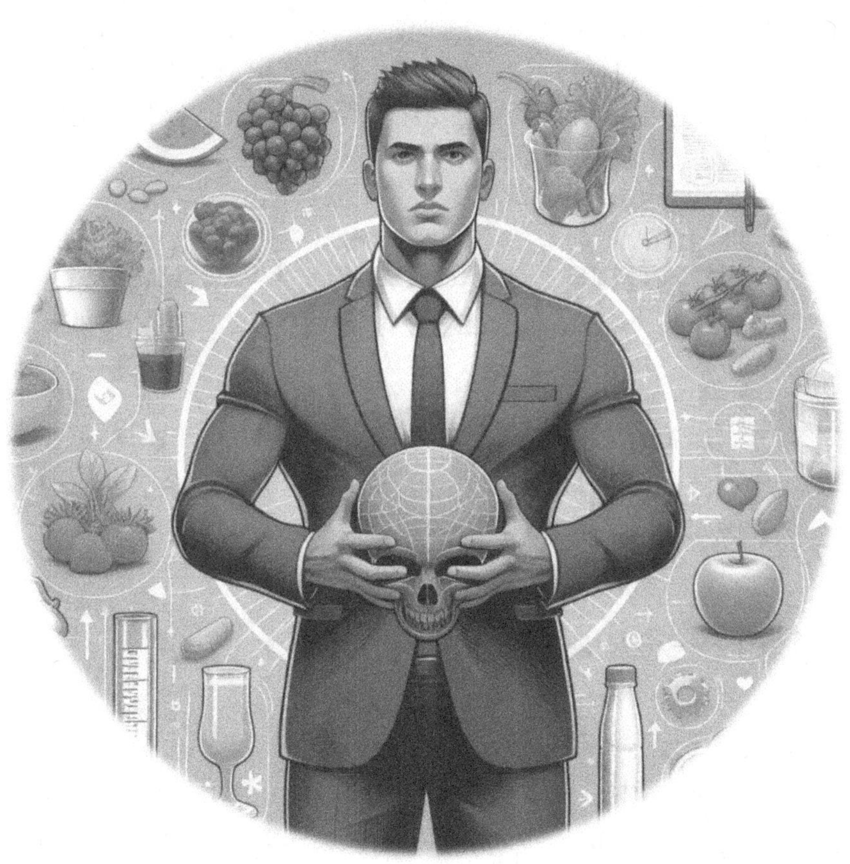

Weight management is a multifaceted process influenced by various factors, including genetics, environment, and lifestyle choices. In this chapter, we'll delve into the complexities of weight management, explore the principles of mindful eating and healthy habits for sustainable weight management, debunk myths surrounding quick fixes and unrealistic weight loss goals, emphasize the importance of focusing on overall health and body composition, and provide actionable steps to develop a personalized plan with sustainable dietary and exercise habits for long-term success.

Factors Influencing Weight Management

Weight management is influenced by a combination of genetic predisposition, environmental factors, and individual lifestyle choices.

Key Influencing Factors:

- Genetics: Genetic factors can influence metabolism, appetite regulation, and body composition, impacting an individual's susceptibility to weight gain or loss.

- Environment: Environmental factors such as food availability, socioeconomic status, cultural norms, and advertising influence dietary choices, physical activity levels, and overall weight status.

- Lifestyle Choices: Diet, physical activity, sleep, stress management, and other lifestyle factors play significant roles in weight management, with small changes accumulating to produce meaningful outcomes over time.

Mindful Eating and Healthy Habits for Sustainable Weight Management

Mindful eating and cultivating healthy habits are essential components of sustainable weight management, focusing on long-term behavior change rather than short-term fixes.

Principles of Mindful Eating:

- Awareness: Pay attention to hunger and satiety cues, eating slowly and mindfully to recognize when you're comfortably full.
- Non-Judgment: Approach food choices without guilt or shame, honoring your body's natural cues and preferences.
- Savoring: Engage all senses while eating, appreciating the flavors, textures, and aromas of your food.
- Self-Compassion: Practice kindness and compassion toward yourself, letting go of

perfectionism and embracing imperfection in your eating habits.

Healthy Habits for Sustainable Weight Management:

- Balanced Diet: Emphasize whole, nutrient-dense foods such as fruits, vegetables, lean proteins, whole grains, and healthy fats, while minimizing processed and refined foods high in added sugars and unhealthy fats.

- Regular Physical Activity: Incorporate regular exercise into your routine, including both aerobic activities (such as walking, jogging, or cycling) and strength training exercises to support muscle mass and metabolism.

- Adequate Sleep: Prioritize quality sleep by maintaining a consistent sleep schedule, creating a restful sleep environment, and practicing relaxation techniques to improve sleep quality and duration.

- Stress Management: Manage stress through relaxation techniques, mindfulness practices, hobbies, and social support, reducing emotional eating and stress-related weight gain.

Debunking Myths Surrounding Quick Fixes and Unrealistic Weight Loss Goals

Despite pervasive myths and misconceptions, there are no quick fixes or magic solutions for sustainable weight management, and unrealistic weight loss goals can be counterproductive and harmful.

Myth: "Diet Pills and Supplements Guarantee Rapid Weight Loss."

Fact: Diet pills and supplements marketed for weight loss often lack scientific evidence and may have adverse side effects. Sustainable weight management requires a balanced diet, regular physical activity, and lifestyle modifications, rather than relying on quick fixes or shortcuts.

Myth: "Losing Weight Quickly is Always Healthy and Sustainable."

Fact: Rapid weight loss can result in muscle loss, nutrient deficiencies, and metabolic slowdown, making it difficult to maintain long-term. Slow, steady weight loss achieved through healthy lifestyle changes is more sustainable and promotes overall health and well-being.

Focusing on Overall Health and Body Composition vs. Weight

Rather than fixating solely on the number on the scale, it's important to focus on overall health, well-being, and body composition when pursuing weight management goals.

Health-Focused Approach:

- Body Composition: Aim to improve body composition by increasing lean muscle mass and reducing excess body fat, rather than focusing solely on weight loss.

- Health Markers: Monitor health markers such as blood pressure, cholesterol levels, blood sugar levels, and waist circumference to assess progress and overall health status.

- Quality of Life: Prioritize behaviors that enhance quality of life, such as improved energy levels, mobility, mood, and self-confidence, rather than solely focusing on weight-related goals.

Action Steps: Developing a Personalized Plan for Sustainable Weight Management

To develop a personalized plan for sustainable weight management, consider the following action steps:

1. Set Realistic Goals: Establish realistic, achievable goals based on your individual preferences, lifestyle, and health status, focusing on gradual progress and long-term success.

2. Create a Balanced Eating Plan: Develop a balanced eating plan that emphasizes whole, nutrient-dense foods and incorporates mindful eating practices to promote satiety and satisfaction.

3. Incorporate Regular Physical Activity: Incorporate regular physical activity into your routine, choosing activities you enjoy and can sustain long-term, such as walking, dancing, swimming, or yoga.

4. Prioritize Sleep and Stress Management: Prioritize adequate sleep and stress management techniques to support overall well-being and reduce the risk of stress-related weight gain.

5. Seek Support and Accountability: Enlist the support of friends, family, or a healthcare professional to provide accountability, encouragement, and guidance on your weight management journey.

Conclusion: Empowering Sustainable Behavior Change for Lifelong Health

In conclusion, sustainable weight management requires a holistic approach that addresses the complex interplay of genetics, environment, and lifestyle factors. By focusing on mindful eating, cultivating healthy habits, and debunking myths surrounding quick fixes and unrealistic goals, you can develop a personalized plan that promotes long-term success and overall well-being. Remember to prioritize overall health and body composition over weight, and celebrate progress in all aspects of your health journey. By taking proactive steps to nurture your physical, emotional, and mental well-being, you can empower yourself to achieve lasting health and vitality for life.

Chapter 14

Nutrition for Different Life Stages

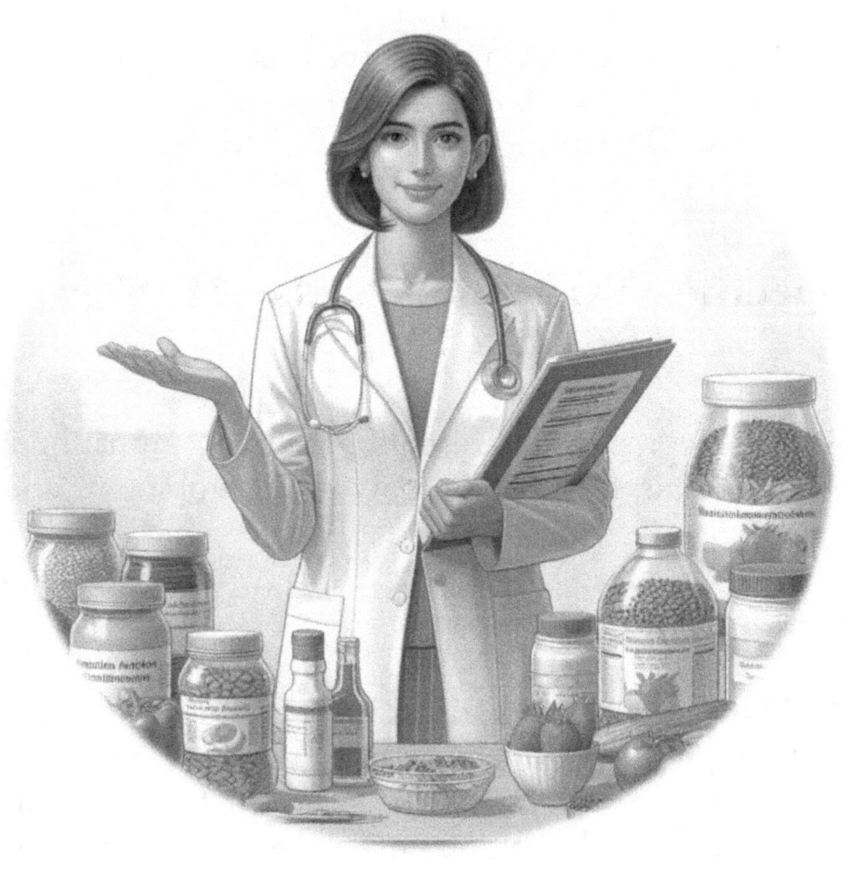

Nutrition plays a critical role in supporting health and well-being throughout various life stages, from infancy to old age. In this chapter, we'll discuss the specific nutritional needs of children, adolescents, pregnant women, and older adults, explore the importance of tailoring your diet to support your body's changing needs, debunk myths surrounding specific diets or restrictions during different life stages, highlight the importance of consulting healthcare professionals for personalized guidance, and provide actionable steps to adapt your dietary patterns and portion sizes according to your age and activity level.

Specific Nutritional Needs of Different Life Stages

Each life stage presents unique nutritional requirements to support growth, development, and overall health.

Children and Adolescents:

- Nutrient-Dense Foods: Children and adolescents need nutrient-dense foods rich in vitamins, minerals, protein, and healthy fats to support growth, development, and academic performance.
- Calcium and Vitamin D: Adequate calcium and vitamin D intake is essential for building strong bones and teeth during childhood and

adolescence.

- Iron: Iron is crucial for cognitive development and oxygen transport in the body, making it essential for growing children and adolescents, especially during periods of rapid growth and development.

Pregnant Women:

- Folate and Iron: Pregnant women require increased folate and iron to support fetal development and prevent neural tube defects and anemia.
- Omega-3 Fatty Acids: Omega-3 fatty acids are important for fetal brain and eye development, making fish rich in omega-3s, such as salmon and sardines, beneficial during pregnancy.
- Protein: Adequate protein intake supports the growth and development of the placenta, fetus, and maternal tissues during pregnancy.

Older Adults:

- Calcium and Vitamin D: Older adults need sufficient calcium and vitamin D to maintain bone health and prevent osteoporosis and fractures.
- Protein: Protein requirements may increase with age to support muscle maintenance, repair, and

function, reducing the risk of sarcopenia and frailty.

- B Vitamins: B vitamins, particularly B12, become more critical as people age, as absorption may decline with age, leading to deficiencies and neurological complications.

Tailoring Your Diet to Support Changing Needs

Adapting your diet to support your body's changing needs throughout life is essential for maintaining health and well-being.

Key Principles for Dietary Adaptation:

- Variety: Include a variety of foods from all food groups to ensure adequate intake of essential nutrients.

- Balance: Balance energy intake with physical activity to maintain a healthy weight and energy balance.

- Moderation: Practice moderation in portion sizes and consumption of foods high in added sugars, unhealthy fats, and sodium.

- Flexibility: Be flexible in your dietary choices, adapting to changing tastes, preferences, and nutritional needs over time.

Debunking Myths Surrounding Specific Diets or Restrictions

There are many myths surrounding specific diets or restrictions during different life stages that may not be supported by scientific evidence.

Myth: "Pregnant Women Should Eat for Two."
Fact: While pregnant women do require additional nutrients, the concept of "eating for two" can lead to excessive weight gain and complications during pregnancy. Instead, focus on nutrient-dense foods and appropriate portion sizes to meet increased nutritional needs.

Myth: "Older Adults Should Avoid Protein to Protect Kidney Health."
Fact: Adequate protein intake is essential for maintaining muscle mass, strength, and function in older adults. While people with kidney disease may need to limit protein intake, most older adults can safely consume moderate amounts of protein as part of a balanced diet.

Importance of Consulting Healthcare Professionals for Personalized Guidance

Consulting healthcare professionals, such as registered dietitians or physicians, is essential for personalized guidance and support tailored to individual needs.

Benefits of Professional Guidance:

Personalization: Healthcare professionals can provide personalized dietary recommendations based on individual health status, medical history, and nutritional needs.

Monitoring and Support: Regular monitoring and support from healthcare professionals can help track progress, make adjustments to dietary plans, and address any concerns or challenges that arise.

Preventing Nutrient Deficiencies: Healthcare professionals can help prevent nutrient deficiencies or imbalances that may occur with certain dietary restrictions or life stages, ensuring overall nutritional adequacy.

Action Steps: Adapting Dietary Patterns According to Age and Activity Level

To adapt your dietary patterns according to your age and activity level, consider the following action steps:

1. Assess Nutritional Needs: Evaluate your individual nutritional needs based on your age, gender, activity level, and life stage, and adjust your dietary intake accordingly.

2. Incorporate Nutrient-Dense Foods: Include a variety of nutrient-dense foods from all food groups in your diet to ensure adequate intake of essential nutrients.

3. Monitor Portion Sizes: Be mindful of portion sizes, adjusting them to match your energy needs and activity level, and avoid excessive calorie intake.

4. Stay Hydrated: Drink plenty of water throughout the day to stay hydrated, particularly during periods of increased physical activity or hot weather.

5. Seek Professional Advice: Consult with a registered dietitian or healthcare provider for personalized guidance and support tailored to your individual needs and goals.

Conclusion: Nurturing Health and Well-being Across the Lifespan

In conclusion, nutrition plays a vital role in supporting health and well-being across various life stages, from childhood to old age. By understanding and addressing the specific nutritional needs of different life stages, adapting dietary patterns accordingly, and debunking myths surrounding specific diets or restrictions, you can optimize health and vitality throughout the lifespan. Remember to prioritize balanced nutrition, regular physical activity, and personalized guidance from healthcare professionals to support overall health and well-being at every stage of life. By taking proactive steps to nurture health and well-being across the lifespan, you can enjoy a vibrant and fulfilling life with optimal health and vitality.

Chapter 15

Food and Culture: Embracing Diversity

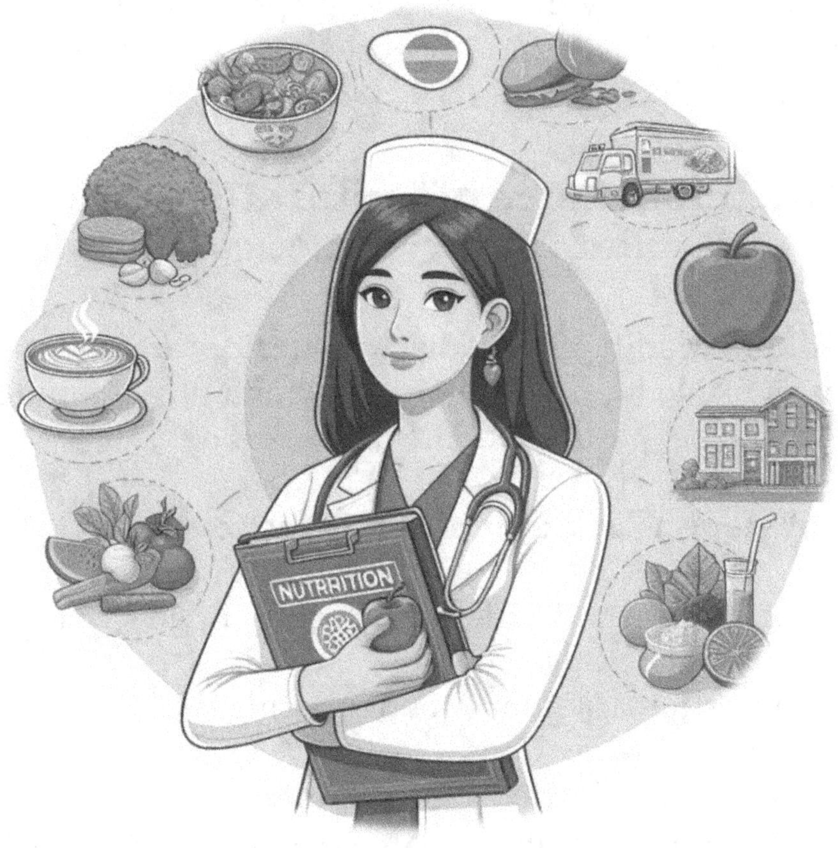

Food is not only sustenance but also a cornerstone of culture, connecting people through shared traditions, flavors, and experiences. In this chapter, we'll discuss the importance of cultural traditions and dietary practices, explore strategies for incorporating healthy adaptations of favorite cultural dishes, highlight the joy of food and its role in fostering connections, debunk myths surrounding cultural foods, and provide actionable steps to learn about the cultural significance of food and embrace culinary diversity.

The Importance of Cultural Traditions and Dietary Practices

Cultural traditions and dietary practices are integral parts of identity, heritage, and community, shaping the way people eat and interact with food.

Key Aspects of Cultural Food Practices:

- Heritage and Identity: Food often reflects cultural heritage, identity, and values, preserving ancestral traditions and passing them down through generations.
- Social Connection: Shared meals and culinary traditions foster social bonds, strengthening relationships and promoting a sense of belonging within communities.
- Celebration and Ritual: Food plays a central role in celebrations, rituals, and religious ceremonies,

marking significant events and bringing people together in shared experiences.

Strategies for Incorporating Healthy Adaptations of Cultural Dishes

While traditional cultural dishes may not always align with current dietary recommendations, there are ways to adapt them to be healthier without sacrificing flavor or authenticity.

Tips for Healthy Adaptations:

- Choose Whole Ingredients: Opt for whole, minimally processed ingredients whenever possible, such as whole grains, lean proteins, and fresh produce, to enhance nutritional quality.
- Modify Cooking Methods: Experiment with healthier cooking methods, such as grilling, baking, or steaming, instead of frying, to reduce added fats and calories.
- Increase Vegetable Content: Incorporate a variety of colorful vegetables into traditional dishes to boost fiber, vitamins, and minerals while adding texture and flavor.
- Reduce Added Sugars and Sodium: Use natural sweeteners sparingly and season dishes with herbs, spices, and citrus juices instead of salt to lower added sugars and sodium content.

Highlighting the Joy of Food and Connection Through Shared Meals

Food has the power to bring people together, fostering joy, connection, and shared experiences around the table.

Benefits of Shared Meals:

- Cultural Exchange: Shared meals provide opportunities for cultural exchange, allowing individuals to learn about and appreciate diverse culinary traditions and flavors.
- Communication and Bonding: Breaking bread together promotes communication, conversation, and bonding, strengthening relationships and building community.
- Cultural Preservation: Sharing traditional dishes and recipes preserves cultural heritage and fosters a sense of pride and connection to one's roots.

Debunking Myths Surrounding Cultural Foods

Despite the richness and diversity of cultural cuisines, there are common misconceptions and stereotypes surrounding certain cultural foods.

Myth: "Cultural Foods Are Unhealthy and Should Be

Avoided."

Fact: Cultural foods are not inherently unhealthy; rather, it's the preparation methods, portion sizes, and frequency of consumption that may influence health outcomes. With mindful choices and healthy adaptations, cultural dishes can be part of a balanced diet.

Myth: "Cultural Foods Need to Be Completely Eliminated for Better Health."

Fact: Restricting or eliminating cultural foods can lead to feelings of deprivation, resentment, and disconnection from one's heritage. Instead, focus on moderation, balance, and mindful eating to enjoy cultural foods while supporting overall health and well-being.

Action Steps: Embracing Culinary Diversity and Cultural Significance

To embrace culinary diversity and honor the cultural significance of food, consider the following action steps:

1. Explore Cultural Foods: Learn about different cultural cuisines, ingredients, and cooking techniques through cookbooks, cooking classes, or cultural festivals.
2. Experiment with Recipes: Try cooking traditional

dishes from diverse cultures, experimenting with healthy adaptations and incorporating new flavors and ingredients into your culinary repertoire.

3. Share Meals with Others: Host multicultural potlucks or dinner parties where guests can bring and share dishes from their cultural backgrounds, promoting cultural exchange and appreciation.

4. Celebrate Food Traditions: Participate in cultural celebrations, festivals, or community events centered around food, honoring traditions and connecting with others through shared culinary experiences.

5. Engage in Dialogue: Engage in conversations about food and culture with friends, family, and colleagues, sharing stories, memories, and recipes that reflect cultural heritage and diversity.

Conclusion: Celebrating Diversity Through Food

In conclusion, food is a universal language that transcends borders, connecting people across cultures, generations, and continents. By embracing culinary diversity, learning about different cultural traditions, and sharing meals with others, we celebrate the richness and beauty of human diversity while fostering understanding, empathy, and connection. Let us debunk myths, break down barriers, and build bridges through the joy of food, honoring cultural heritage, and savoring the flavors of our shared humanity. Together, we can create a world where food is not only nourishment but also a source of unity, celebration, and love.

CONCLUSION

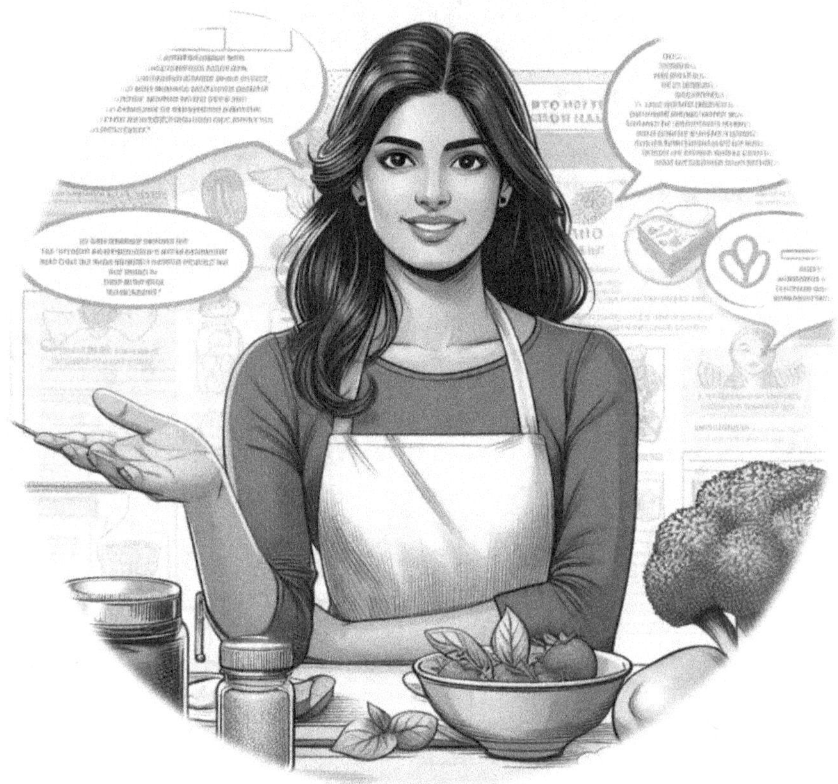

Throughout this book, we've embarked on a journey to debunk diet myths and explore the principles of responsible eating for optimal health and happiness. As we come to the end of our exploration, let's recap the key takeaways and reiterate the importance of adopting a personalized and sustainable approach to nutrition.

Key Takeaways:

1. Evidence-Based Eating: Instead of falling for fad diets or quick fixes, prioritize evidence-based nutrition by focusing on whole, minimally processed foods and listening to your body's cues.

2. Macronutrient Balance: Understand the roles of carbohydrates, proteins, and fats in your diet, and tailor your macronutrient intake to support your activity level and goals.

3. Micronutrient Sufficiency: Ensure you're meeting your body's needs for essential vitamins and minerals by consuming a diverse array of fruits, vegetables, whole grains, and lean proteins.

4. Gut Health and Digestion: Support gut health and digestion by incorporating probiotic-rich foods, fiber, and mindful eating practices into your daily routine.

5. Mindful Eating: Practice mindful eating to reconnect with your body's hunger and satiety cues, savor your food, and cultivate a positive relationship with eating.

6. Balanced Plate: Build balanced meals using MyPlate or similar models, incorporating a

variety of food groups to ensure a diverse and nutrient-rich diet.

7. Healthy Habits: Embrace healthy lifestyle habits such as regular physical activity, adequate hydration, stress management, and quality sleep to support overall well-being.

Personalized and Sustainable Approach:

Remember, there's no one-size-fits-all approach to nutrition. It's essential to tailor your eating patterns to your individual needs, preferences, and goals, taking into account factors such as age, gender, activity level, and health status. By adopting a personalized and sustainable approach to nutrition, you can achieve long-term success and maintain a healthy relationship with food.

Seeking Professional Guidance:

For personalized guidance and support, consider consulting with a registered dietitian or healthcare professional. They can provide tailored recommendations, address specific dietary concerns or conditions, and help you navigate the wealth of nutrition information available.

Empowerment and Informed Choices:

As you close this book, I hope you feel empowered and equipped to make informed choices about your health and well-being. Armed with evidence-based knowledge, practical tips, and a deeper understanding of nutrition, you have the tools to cultivate a lifestyle that nourishes your body, mind, and soul.

Remember, every meal is an opportunity to nourish yourself and honor your body's needs. By embracing responsible eating practices, debunking diet myths, and celebrating the joy of food, you're on the path to optimal health and happiness.

Here's to your journey towards a life filled with vitality, balance, and well-being. Cheers to a future where you thrive, fueled by the wisdom of informed choices and the joy of nourishing food.

ABOUT THE AUTHOR

Adeel Anjum is a visionary business leader with an illustrious career spanning over 20 years in strategic management and consulting. With a dynamic background that includes diverse industries such as sports retail, fashion retail, food retail, oil & gas, F&B, fitness & leisure, as well as technology & telecom retail, Adeel has amassed a wealth of experience and expertise in driving organizational success.

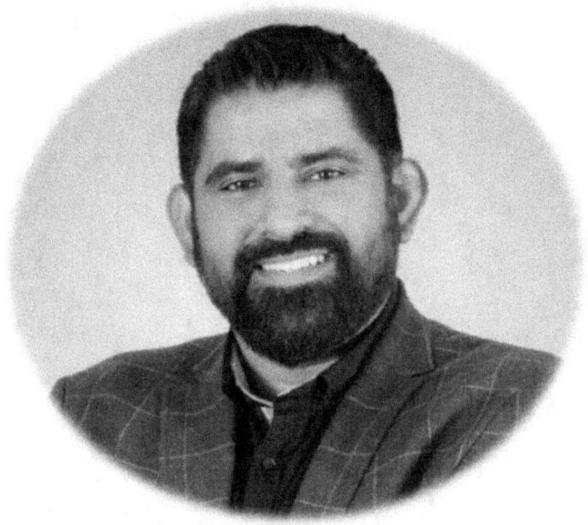

As a thought leader, Adeel Anjum stands at the forefront of shaping the business community through his pioneering work, insightful writings, and groundbreaking research. With a commitment to innovation and a deep understanding of Industry dynamics, Adeel Anjum inspires and guides fellow professionals, fostering a culture of continuous learning and strategic evolution within the business landscape.

Driven by a steadfast commitment to contribute to the business world, I am channeling my knowledge and experience into meaningful narratives within my books. My aim is to offer valuable insights, lessons, and strategies that empower individuals and organizations. Through the written word, I aspire to give back to the business community, sharing the wisdom gained on my journey and inspiring others to achieve their fullest potential and mindfulness..